The ABCs of CBM

The Guilford Practical Intervention in the Schools Series

Kenneth W. Merrell, Founding Editor
Sandra M. Chafouleas, Series Editor

www.guilford.com/practical

This series presents the most reader-friendly resources available in key areas of evidence-based practice in school settings. Practitioners will find trustworthy guides on effective behavioral, mental health, and academic interventions, and assessment and measurement approaches. Covering all aspects of planning, implementing, and evaluating high-quality services for students, books in the series are carefully crafted for everyday utility. Features include ready-to-use reproducibles, appealing visual elements, and an oversized format. Recent titles have Web pages where purchasers can download and print the reproducible materials.

Recent Volumes

Assessing Intelligence in Children and Adolescents: A Practical Guide
John H. Kranzler and Randy G. Floyd

The RTI Approach to Evaluating Learning Disabilities
Joseph F. Kovaleski, Amanda M. VanDerHayden, and Edward S. Shapiro

Resilient Classrooms, Second Edition:
Creating Healthy Environments for Learning
Beth Doll, Katherine Brehm, and Steven Zucker

The ABCs of Curriculum-Based Evaluation:
A Practical Guide to Effective Decision Making
John L. Hosp, Michelle K. Hosp, Kenneth W. Howell, and Randy Allison

Curriculum-Based Assessment for Instructional Design:
Using Data to Individualize Instruction
Matthew K. Burns and David C. Parker

Dropout Prevention
C. Lee Goss and Kristina J. Andren

Stress Management for Teachers: A Proactive Guide
Keith C. Herman and Wendy M. Reinke

Interventions for Reading Problems, Second Edition:
Designing and Evaluating Effective Strategies
*Edward J. Daly III, Sabina Neugebauer, Sandra Chafouleas,
and Christopher H. Skinner*

Classwide Positive Behavior Interventions and Supports:
A Guide to Proactive Classroom Management
Brandi Simonsen and Diane Myers

Promoting Academic Success with English Language Learners: Best Practices for RTI
Craig A. Albers and Rebecca S. Martinez

Integrated Multi-Tiered Systems of Support: Blending RTI and PBIS
Kent McIntosh and Steve Goodman

The ABCs of CBM, Second Edition:
A Practical Guide to Curriculum-Based Measurement
Michelle K. Hosp, John L. Hosp, and Kenneth W. Howell

The ABCs of CBM

A Practical Guide
to Curriculum-Based Measurement

SECOND EDITION

MICHELLE K. HOSP
JOHN L. HOSP
KENNETH W. HOWELL

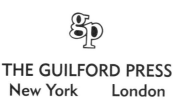

THE GUILFORD PRESS
New York   London

Copyright © 2016 The Guilford Press
A Division of Guilford Publications, Inc.
370 Seventh Avenue, Suite 1200, New York, NY 10001
www.guilford.com

Printed in the United States of America

This book is printed on acid-free paper.

Last digit is print number: 9   8   7   6   5   4

Library of Congress Cataloging-in-Publication Data

Names: Hosp, Michelle K. | Hosp, John L. | Howell, Kenneth W.
Title: The ABCs of CBM : a practical guide to curriculum-based measurement /
    Michelle K. Hosp, John L. Hosp, Kenneth W. Howell.
Description: Second edition. | New York : The Guilford Press, 2016. | Series:
    The Guilford practical intervention in the schools series | Includes
    bibliographical references and index.
Identifiers: LCCN 2015051242 | ISBN 9781462524662 (paperback)
Subjects: LCSH: Curriculum-based assessment—United States. | Educational
    tests and measurements—United States. | BISAC: PSYCHOLOGY / Psychotherapy
    / Child & Adolescent. | EDUCATION / Special Education / General. | MEDICAL
    / Psychiatry / Child & Adolescent. | SOCIAL SCIENCE / Social Work.
Classification: LCC LB3060.32.C74 H67 2016 | DDC 375/.006—dc23
LC record available at *http://lccn.loc.gov/2015051242*

To all who are reading this
—DANIEL HOSP

About the Authors

Michelle K. Hosp, PhD, is Associate Professor of Special Education at the University of Massachusetts Amherst. A nationally known trainer and speaker on problem solving and the use of progress monitoring data, she has served as Director of the Iowa Reading Research Center and as a trainer with the National Center on Progress Monitoring and the National Center on Response to Intervention, and is currently on the technical review committee for the National Center on Intensive Intervention. Dr. Hosp's research focuses on reading and on multi-tiered systems of support/response to intervention (MTSS/RTI) in relation to curriculum-based measurement (CBM) and curriculum-based evaluation (CBE). She has published numerous articles, book chapters, and books.

John L. Hosp, PhD, is Professor of Special Education at the University of Massachusetts Amherst. His research focuses on MTSS/RTI, including disproportionate representation of minority students in special education and aligning assessment and instruction, particularly in the areas of CBM and CBE. Dr. Hosp has conducted workshops nationally and has authored over 50 journal articles, book chapters, and books. He is coauthor (with Michelle K. Hosp, Kenneth W. Howell, and Randy Allison) of *The ABCs of Curriculum-Based Evaluation.*

Kenneth W. Howell, PhD, is Professor Emeritus of Special Education at Western Washington University. A former general and special education teacher and school psychologist, Dr. Howell's primary focus throughout his career has been on students with learning problems and behavioral difficulties, including adjudicated youth. He has presented nationally and internationally on CBE, MTSS/RTI, juvenile corrections, and social skills, and has published extensively in the areas of CBE, CBM, and problem solving.

Contents

3. How to Conduct Early Reading CBM   **32**

4. How to Conduct Reading CBM   **70**

CHAPTER 1

What Is CBM
and Why Should I Do It?

This book is about an assessment tool called *curriculum-based measurement* (CBM). The book begins by explaining a little bit about what CBM is and where it came from, but the majority of it will focus on the nuts and bolts (i.e., the ABCs) of how to use CBM in a classroom, school, or district to improve the quality of educational decision making.

Given the number of assessment and evaluation initiatives present in education today, you might be wondering why you need to know about CBM. That is a legitimate question.

The main thing we want you to know is that CBM is not something *additional* to do. CBM is an *alternative* to other procedures you may already be doing (or avoiding because they are time consuming or too complex to justify). Time spent assessing often takes time away from teaching—particularly if the methods are inefficient or unrelated to instruction and improved student outcomes.

Imagine that you are planning a trip and you need to drive somewhere. You have your choice of many different schedules and routes. So you decide to check the "Traditional Assessment" travel agency website. When you pull up the web page there is a list of roads between your home and your destination. With no place to enter information about where you're starting or where you're going, you can't plan a route (destinations like "in California" aren't all that helpful).

So, you try CBM Travel. The CBM page begins by asking for explicit information about your current location and your destination. It also asks exactly where you want to end up and when you want to be there. Also, CBM Travel comes with a service that monitors your progress and, by immediately noting if you get off your original route, tells you when to adjust the path you're traveling. This way you don't get further behind and will make up the time you've lost! Our guess is you will ditch Traditional Assessment Travel and go for CBM!

Here are the things you need to know about CBM before you head out:

1. CBM is not an "add-on"; CBM is an alternative. You wouldn't make your trip twice, once with Traditional Assessment Travel *and* once with CBM Travel. Why would you assess twice to make one decision?
2. CBM is a bargain. CBM gets you where you are going by helping you improve student learning in less time and with less cost.

WHY DO I NEED THIS BOOK?

This book includes a set of skills that lead to quality instruction. It is about collecting and using information. Whenever we work at something important, it is best to develop a plan before we start and to check on our progress while we are working. This allows us to work in an intentional and thoughtful way. It defines what we are trying to accomplish, alerts us when what we are doing isn't getting us closer to that goal, and gives us the information we need to determine how to change. Educating children, adolescents, and young adults certainly fits within the definition of an important activity. Therefore the process of education should include things like goal setting, planning, instruction, and monitoring. To do these things well, an educator needs information! The quality of the information you have will determine the quality of the work you do.

In the United States, for example, there are literally millions of school-age students with serious reading problems. These include students coming from low-income families or belonging to certain linguistic or racial/ethnic groups. As a result, educators have an increased responsibility to make informed decisions when working to teach important skills like reading and when tackling the needs of students who face problems learning. But it is difficult for teachers to think their way through these important efforts without something concrete to think about. CBM provides exactly the kind of functional information required to inform educational decision making. Therefore this book is designed to teach you how to get and use that information.

WHAT IS CBM?

CBM is an assessment tool characterized by certain attributes. We'll explain these attributes shortly, but first you should know what CBM "looks" like.

CBM is usually composed of a set of standardized directions, a timing device, a set of materials (i.e., passages, sheets, lists), scoring rules, standards for judging performance, and record forms or charts. The directions given are very straightforward in that they ask the student to engage in a task that is not that different than something she would do during class (e.g., read from a book, write a paragraph, or solve computation problems). The materials the student works on will look just like class materials. During CBM, as the student performs these tasks you'll see that she is timed so that her level of performance can be scored in terms of the number of responses correct and incorrect per minute (e.g., "Student reads

47 words correctly and 8 incorrectly in 1 minute"). Therefore the person giving the test will have some sort of timer. Also, you will probably see the student's level of performance on curriculum-based measures charted on a graph or entered into a computer so that trends in her learning can be analyzed over time.

When watching CBM, because you won't see the performance standards or the scoring rules being used; you might not even recognize the administration of the curriculum-based measures as a test or assessment. It will look very much like a teaching activity (except without the corrective feedback). That is because one of the supporting principles of CBM is an idea called *alignment*. The principle of alignment basically holds that your educational efforts will be more effective if you "test what you teach and teach what you test." *What* you teach is called the *curriculum*. It is the goals and objectives that must be met to achieve social and academic competence. (This is a fairly standard definition. The word *curriculum* comes from the Latin word *currer* for racing chariots. The curriculum, then, is the "course of study" to be followed on the way to the finish line.)

WHY WERE THE OTHER ATTRIBUTES, LIKE THE TIMING AND CHARTING, DEVELOPED?

CBM evolved out of work by Stan Deno and Phyllis Mirkin in the late 1970s and early 1980s at the Minnesota Institute for Research on Learning Disabilities (Deno & Mirkin, 1977). They were working on an intervention process called data-based program modification (DBPM). DBPM was a complete package of procedures for establishing goals, planning interventions (with a heavy emphasis on collaboration and consultation), and monitoring. However, in order for DBPM to work, there needed to be a continuous data collection system in place to produce the information needed to guide the decisions that fueled the program modifications. It was also needed because, as many of the instructional interventions were designed through consultation, the person delivering the lessons was not always the person responsible for the students' learning (just like today).

Deno and Mirkin realized that they needed an assessment system built on a set of common principles and composed of standardized procedures and rules. In a way, this sort of system already existed in the form of applied behavior analysis for areas such as classroom management and social behavior. But there wasn't a system like that for academic content. So Deno and Mirkin began developing CBM.

CBM is characterized by several attributes (Deno, 2003):

1. The first and most obvious is *alignment*. Within CBM the students are tested on the curriculum they are being taught. This means:

- The content is the same;
- The stimulus materials the student is given look the same; and
- The responses she is expected to make are the same.

2. The measures are *technically adequate*. This means they must have established reliability and validity. For evidence of the reliability and validity of many curriculum-

based measures, you can check out the National Center on Intensive Intervention (NCII) for progress monitoring (*www.intensiveintervention.org*) and the Center on Response to Intervention for screening (*www.rti4success.org*). Even though CBM is used within classrooms by teachers, it is *not* informal assessment! "Informal assessments" typically have not been shown to be technically adequate (that's one of the things that makes them informal, not a tendency for the assessor to wear jeans and a T-shirt).

CBM is an empirically supported process with substantial technical adequacy. Over the past 30 years, there have been hundreds of solid empirical research studies in excellent journals supporting the application of CBM. In fact, because CBM is used to summarize both a student's level of performance and her rate of progress, it has been examined in ways traditional measures have never been examined.

3. CBM typically makes use of *criterion-referenced standards* as opposed to norm-referenced standards (we'll explain this later).

4. *Standardized procedures* are used for administering and scoring curriculum-based measures. All those using CBM who want to share their data with others (e.g., as part of a program evaluation or a formal student report) must follow the same administration and scoring rules. For example:

- Standard tasks are used for each content area (e.g., three 1-minute timed oral readings are used to find a student's current level of reading performance);
- Standard procedures are followed for selecting or constructing testing materials; and
- Standard administration and scoring directions are employed for each procedure.

5. *Performance sampling* is used (producing what is sometimes called *behavioral data*). CBM procedures employ direct, *low-inference* measures through which correct and incorrect student behaviors, on clearly defined tasks, are counted within a set time interval (usually in minutes). Therefore, inference and conjecture about the meaning of the resulting scores is kept to a minimum. For example, a reading CBM might tell you that the student read a fifth-grade-level passage at "47 words correct per minute with no errors."

6. Decision rules are put in place to provide those who use the data with information about what it means when students score at different levels of performance or illustrate different rates of progress on the measures over time. These rules are based on performance criteria and standardized through sampling or experimental procedures.

7. CBM emphasizes *repeated measurement* over time and can be used to identify *rates of progress* as well as *levels of performance*. Therefore, CBM data can be used for *progress monitoring* to examine learning *as it is occurring*. This allows teachers to make immediate adjustments in a student's educational program when needed. Because CBM also measures what is being taught, and learning is a change in performance over time, these repeated measures illustrate the degree to which current instructional interventions are producing learning. As a result, the use of CBM and progress monitoring allows educators to judge the quality of their own instruction (and to decide when changes need to be made). Therefore, CBM data don't just help teachers decide *what* to teach, they can also help them decide *how* to teach.

8. CBM is also *efficient*. It is efficient in implementation because people can be trained to give the measures in a short period of time and the measures can be given quickly. When you use performance data, you draw conclusions directly from what the student actually did on the test. (All educational and psychological measures require students to engage in behavior, but in many cases the original behavior, which is usually called the *raw score*, needs to be converted into another form before it can be used.) There is no need to convert the raw score for most purposes.

For example, if a student reads 47 words per minute and the criterion for this passage is 60 words per minute, then the conclusion is that she is reading 13 words per minute slower than she should. That's it!

For classroom purposes, CBM results are summarized and interpreted as simple performance statements and do not need to be converted into percentiles or normal-curve equivalents to be understood. All you need to know is that the student reading 47 words correctly per minute must be taught to read 13 words per minute faster than she is currently.

9. Last, the CBM data can be *summarized efficiently* by using a variety of techniques ranging from pencil-and-paper charts to a web-based data management system. This efficiency makes the data immediately accessible at any level of the educational system. Most important, it makes the data accessible to classroom teachers and students!

WHY IS CBM DIFFERENT FROM OTHER FORMS OF MEASUREMENT?

Many of the most important differences were spelled out in the nine attributes listed above. However, there are some fundamental CBM ideas that support those attributes.

Anyone who has spent time around education knows that there are all kinds of assessments available in schools. These range in structure from statewide accountability tests to simple handwriting rubrics. In education, we use these measures to inform our decision making. And the forms of these measures usually have to do with the functions they are designed to fulfill.

There are different forms of measures because there are different kinds of decisions to make and different ways to go about making decisions. CBM, as explained above, was designed to help teachers plan instruction and monitor outcomes to see if instruction is working. There are four ways the structures of CBM reflect this purpose: (1) by aligning with the *curriculum*; (2) by measuring *alterable variables*; (3) by employing *low-inference measures*; and (4) by employing *criterion-referenced* measures.

Curriculum

When we say a measure is curriculum-based, we expect to see that measure sampling the things that students are taught. This might not be the case for measures based on ideas about general achievement, disability type, learning style, fixed ability (e.g., intelligence or cognitive ability), developmental stages, or perceptual processing. Those tests may not be built to target the content a student is being taught. In fact, they may actually have been written to avoid it.

Our guess is that you anticipated curriculum-based measures reflecting the curriculum (good for you!). But CBM is also designed to function within instructional systems that include systematic instructional interventions and student mastery of performance goals (such as a multi-tiered system of supports [MTSS] also called response to intervention [RTI] frameworks). That kind of system needs direct measurement of student learning to function. Measures designed to function in other problem-solving paradigms, such as the traditional student-deficit model or those that assume that instruction should yield a normal distribution of skills, are designed differently. But how are they different?

Alterable Variables

One of the most important differences between CBM and other measures used in education and psychology is that CBM targets alterable variables. In education, an *alterable variable* is something that can be changed *through instruction.* Performance on curricular tasks is considered alterable because it is under the direct control of teachers (i.e., student performance can be changed through effective instruction). CBM was not designed simply to document the existence of problems or even to determine their cause. It was designed as a data collection system that would produce the information required to guide instruction. One of the things CBM can do very well, for example, is tell a teacher about the level of a student's knowledge about a particular skill. This information has immediate implications for instruction because instruction, by definition, is the provision of new knowledge.

This brings us to the issue of alterable and unalterable variables. There is considerable debate about whether measures of unalterable student-centered variables (like perceptual processing, developmental stage, learning style, or even IQ level) provide useful information for guiding instruction. More to the point, the status of a student's curricular skills *can* be changed by the teacher through instruction. However, things like learning style, cognitive ability, and even general achievement are traditionally conceptualized as being relatively stable. As a consequence, time spent measuring them, assuming the measures work, is time spent looking at things that teachers can't do anything about. Worse yet, even if measures of those variables work, the information they yield is still useless without good information about what skills a student needs to learn—so, in the end, CBM is always needed.

Low-Inference Measures

Tools that measure one thing so that conclusions can be drawn about something else require us to make *inferences.* Those that require us to process assessment results by way of some theoretical application are called *high-inference* measures. For example, a cognitive ability test (e.g., IQ test) does not have any cognitive ability items on it, but it does have items from which the test user is expected to make *inferences* about the student's cognitive ability. Therefore, while a student may assemble geometric shapes out of blocks on a cognitive ability test, the score is not reported in terms of "geometric shape production," but in terms of "cognitive ability." We can only accept such interpretations if we accept the theory of cognitive ability on which the inference is based.

The fact that CBM is designed to sample the observable student behaviors that occur in a classroom distinguishes it sharply from the high-inference measures often used in education and school psychology. CBM was not developed to explain how learning does or doesn't occur. And it was not designed to conform to any particular theory about how students think, attend, remember, or process information. Therefore, inference and conjecture about what the resulting scores actually mean is kept to a minimum. Curriculum-based measures employ direct (low-inference) observations during which correct and incorrect student responses to the tasks being taught (e.g., addition) are counted within a set time interval (usually in minutes). If the student works seven addition fact problems in 1 minute, her score is reported as "seven addition facts per minute." If the criterion for addition facts is 40 per minute, the seven-per-minute score is simple to interpret: It means this student needs instruction on addition!

Criterion-Referenced Measures

Another way that CBM is different from most traditional educational and psychological measures is that it escapes the normative tradition and employs criterion-referenced standards (although norms for many of the measures are also available). Criterion-referenced standards are used to determine if students can demonstrate their knowledge of certain tasks at specified performance levels (i.e., criteria). The basic assumption is that students who do not know a skill and need instruction on it will do poorly on the test of that skill. Whereas, those who *do* know the skill will pass the test.

One of the biggest problems with the utility of educational evaluation is that its history has been grounded almost exclusively in *normative standards*. There is nothing wrong with normative comparisons or the measures used to conduct them as long as your goal is to find out how a student's level of performance compares to the performance of others. But that isn't the most important thing teachers need to know! For planning a lesson, it is more important to know if the student has or hasn't mastered the skills about to be covered (or what she needs to be taught next). Knowing how a student compares to other students does not provide that information!

CBM came directly out of an intervention program and was designed to inform teachers' decisions about *what* and *how* to teach. As has already been explained, CBM was designed for instructional utility. This meant that the measures had to be:

- Aligned with curriculum;
- Sensitive to instruction;
- Repeatable so that progress monitoring could occur; and
- Criterion-referenced so that they could be used to determine when a student had mastered a task.

These conditions allow teachers to set goals, determine the level of a student's prerequisite knowledge, align instruction with outcomes, and track progress toward goals.

WHAT ARE THE MAIN ADVANTAGES OF CBM?

If we have to pick a few advantages, we will go with efficiency, alignment, and usefulness in progress monitoring. The first one, efficiency, is important because no one is going to use a measure that is awkward, confusing, or burdensome. CBM is actually quite simple to use and to understand. This means less time assessing and more time teaching.

The second choice would have to be CBM's *alignment*, or linkage, with instructional outcomes. Alignment between measurement and the curriculum being taught allows the user to make better decisions. For example, alignment improves decisions about what the student can and can't do. As you will see, CBM lets us be very precise when selecting instructional goals and determining current levels of performance.

Alignment is often lost with traditional normative measures as these are constructed by using a sample of items selected across a wide range of difficulty. (You're familiar with this format. It is the one that starts with very easy items and moves quickly through increasingly complex material.) Unfortunately, in order to cover a range of skills and keep such tests down to a manageable size, the *curricular distance* between items on these tests is often large, and very few items are provided for each skill. Alignment is lost because of the limited number of items for each skill and because some skills must be completely left off the test.

Alignment is also lost when measures use item formats presenting the student with tasks different from those he actually needs to use. For example, group-administered tests often ask students to identify answers by circling or matching them. In actual practice, students don't need to identify correct answers; they need to produce them! The two skills are different.

Our third choice is CBM's usefulness for progress monitoring. Typical normative achievement measures can't be used to decide if instruction is working within a fairly short period of time. They are designed to yield scores that are highly stable over time (a student's score on normative tests should not change across short periods), and they don't have a sufficient number of alternate forms for frequent retesting. However, CBM allows for progress monitoring by using equivalent samples in a repeated (even daily) measurement format. Frequent use coupled with alignment makes CBM more sensitive to instruction than typical achievement measures. This means it can be used to decide, within a fairly short period of time, when instruction is (or isn't) working. That means CBM can also be used to help one decide *how* to teach. It does this by letting us see, in a timely manner, if the instruction is working and/or when it should be changed.

By opening up access to progress data, CBM supplies educators with a whole new assembly of information. Given that information, they can make a whole new set of informed decisions. Information collected during the process of instruction is called *formative evaluation*. Formative evaluation was a central component of the DBPM system originally developed by Deno and Mirkin. It involves the use of information from repeated direct measures to display trends in learning so that instructional decisions can be based on levels of student progress. This is, hands down, the most powerful tool available to any teacher or school psychologist!

WHAT KINDS OF DECISIONS
CAN I MAKE WITH CBM DATA?

As will be explained in Chapter 2, there are four major kinds of decisions we make in education:

1. *Universal screening decisions* to decide which students need help and which don't;
2. *Progress monitoring decisions* to decide when to move on to new goals or modify instruction;
3. *Diagnostic decisions* to decide what kind of help a student needs; and
4. *Outcome decisions* to decide when special services can be discontinued and to document the overall effectiveness of efforts across all students.

The kinds of measures we use and the ways we use them depend on which kind of decision we are trying to make. As will be explained shortly, *general outcome* and *skills-based* CBMs are often used as survey measures and *mastery measure* CBMs are often used as specific measures.

HOW DOES CBM RELATE
TO MTSS OR RTI?

MTSS and RTI are terms that are often used interchangeably and often mean different things to different people. In general they include the use of data-based decision making for problem solving. Key components of any good MTSS/RTI approach are the use of assessment for universal screening and progress monitoring decisions, provision of instruction and intervention in a tiered system, such that individuals who have greater instructional needs are receiving more instruction and support. As mentioned above (and in more depth in Chapter 2), CBM is an excellent way to make universal screening and progress-monitoring decisions such as those central to MTSS/RTI.

HOW DOES CBM RELATE
TO CURRICULUM-BASED EVALUATION?

The third key component of MTSS/RTI that we mentioned has to do with detailed decision making about student needs and learning. It is a hallmark of MTSS/RTI because students who are experiencing the greatest difficulties are the ones who need the most intensive teaching. Curriculum-based evaluation (CBE) is one approach to instructional decision making to meet the needs of students who are struggling. As you might have guessed from the whole "curriculum-based" thing, CBE is a systematic problem-solving process that relies heavily on CBM for the data on which we base our decisions (i.e., data-based decision making).

SO, CBM DOES JUST ABOUT EVERYTHING?

Well, it doesn't teach!

CBM is *not* an instructional method or intervention. It is a tool for improving instruction that is compatible with diverse instructional approaches. Similarly, CBM is *not* a curriculum. So there isn't a CBM reading program.

CBM is a measurement overlay, which means the CBM administration and scoring rules are like templates that can be laid over goals and objectives from an assortment of content areas. This makes CBM uniquely valuable in situations where different teachers may be using different instructional methods or the same teacher may have different students being taught in different ways.

There are sets of published curriculum-based measures that have been developed around particular sequences of goals, but the tasks and goal sequences used in those measures are not the defining elements of CBM (they are defining elements of the different tasks, objectives, and curriculums on which they are based). The defining elements of CBM are the curriculum-based procedures for designing, administering, and scoring measures as well as recording, summarizing, and interpreting the data that result from those measures. Therefore, you can't buy one CBM that will be useful for all subject areas or in all classrooms.

ARE THERE DIFFERENT TYPES OF CBM?

A measure gets to be a CBM instrument if it is designed, administered, and scored according to established CBM procedures. Three types of CBM procedures have been described: general outcome measures, skills-based measures, and mastery measures. These all share the qualities listed above but may differ in design according to their purposes and the nature of the skills they are designed to test.

General Outcome Measures

General outcome measures (GOMs) are used to sample performance across several goals at the same time by using capstone tasks that are complex in the sense that they can only be accomplished by successfully applying a number of contributing skills. In this measurement format, the contributing skills (i.e., subskills) are not separated out for direct attention as they are in the skills-based measures and mastery measures we'll describe shortly. Instead, success or improvement on the GOM is assumed to reflect the synthetic application of the contributing skills. In this sense, GOMs are holistic, while mastery measures in particular, are atomistic.

Probably the best example of a GOM is oral passage reading. In order for a student to be able to read proficiently, she must be able to use a variety of skills at the same time. Those include the skills required to use letters, letter combinations, blending, vocabulary, syntax, and content knowledge. As a student improves in any of these skills you can expect to see some improvement in her oral passage reading. As a result, using oral reading as the GOM relieves you of the need to monitor each of these subskills separately (whether they are taught in isolation or in combination).

There are several obvious advantages to GOMs. The first is that they dramatically cut down on the number of different measures one has to introduce, manage, administer, score, and track. Having four or five GOMs to cover the areas addressed throughout a year, a teacher can have her monitoring system for the whole year in place on the first day. The use of GOMs also recognizes the limitations of isolating subskills from the context in which they normally are expected to function. Any time you present tasks in a format that is different from the way they will usually be used (e.g., asking students to read nonsense words or the sounds of letters in isolation), there is the risk that you will lose validity. A final advantage is that visual displays of progress on a GOM will show longer acquisition slopes, allowing adequate opportunities for progress monitoring and data-based instructional modifications.

For the reasons listed above, GOMs are especially useful for universal screening and progress monitoring to get an overview of level of performance. The primary disadvantage of GOMs is the downside of all general procedures: they are *general.* If your student's oral reading is inadequate and you think you need specific information about her relative skill patterns, you may not get that information from a GOM. Another limitation of GOMs is that some curriculum areas do not have a capstone task that represents the synthetic application of most of the content (especially one that is reasonably convenient to use). For example, GOMs are difficult to develop in mathematics beyond the early grades.

Skills-Based Measures

Skills-based measures (SBMs) are designed to accomplish many of the functions of GOMs. They also have their particular advantages and disadvantages. Their main advantages are that they can be used to screen and progress monitor in curriculum domains where capstone tasks are not available.

The best example of an SBM is probably math computation. At any particular grade level, a math curriculum for computation is made up of a list of specific skills. For example, a second-grade curriculum might include addition facts, double-digit addition without regrouping, double-digit addition with regrouping, and subtraction facts. There is no single task to demonstrate proficiency on all of these skills—each needs to be measured directly, using an SBM.

SBMs are constructed by first identifying the set of goals that will be taught within a curriculum area. The time frame you will cover could sample goals for an entire year or for shorter periods. Once the goals have been identified, items are then prepared to assess each goal. The items for the same goal should be of equal difficulty. Next, the items are placed in random order (from the student's perspective) into a set of tests (in fact, they should be in a deliberate order, but one that is not readily identifiable). This produces a set of equivalent measures providing balanced coverage of the same content.

The items on these tests are not placed in the order in which they are taught or in order of complexity. All of the items covering the same goal are not grouped together. Items should be arranged so that each goal is equally represented in each section (i.e., beginning, middle, and end) of the test. It is good to note what skills each item is measuring, however, so that you can link performance on the measure back to instructional objectives.

SBMs are generally administered by including directions like "Work as many items as you can. If you come to one you don't know, you can skip it." When given these directions and measures constructed as we have described them, students who are beginning to work on a set of skills will skip many problems and get lower scores. As they progress through the curriculum and learn new skills, their scores will improve because there will be more items they can work. Therefore, SBMs can sometimes be used to progress monitor, as they will produce long acquisition slopes like GOMs do. In addition, they can yield some analytical information as long as steps are taken to ensure that an adequate sample of each kind of item is provided and that the items are cross-referenced to goals.

One big disadvantage of SBMs is that when instruction begins, most of the items will be irrelevant to the student because they will be above her current level of performance. Near the end of instruction, most of the items will again be irrelevant because she will have already learned them. Basically, this means that at any given time only a few items on the test will be directly related to what the student is currently learning.

Mastery Measures

The last type of CBM is the mastery measure (MM). MMs differ from GOMs and SBMs in several ways, mainly in the relative levels within the curriculum from which tasks are drawn and the relative sizes of the measurement net they spread. (The term *measurement net* refers to the size and nature of the sample a measure collects. For example, a test covering 25 computation skills would be casting a larger measurement net than one covering five skills.) GOMs present tasks that are relatively more complex and/or advanced than do MMs; SBMs tend to cover more skills than MMs (i.e., they measure more by casting a wider net). Therefore, MMs are generally used on parts of the curriculum that contain discrete and easily identified sets (or domains) of items that are closely related by some common skill, theme, concept, or solution strategy. Examples of this sort of domain might include punctuation (for writing), multiplying fractions (for math), or sounds of letters (for early reading).

MMs are used in three situations:

1. When you really want to focus on a particular set of skills. These might include the so-called *tool skills*, which need to be performed at high levels of proficiency (e.g., letter formation, using the silent *e* to convert vowels, computation facts). Focus might also be important for skills that are pivotal to many other operations, like quickly going through the steps of multiplying fractions;
2. When you are trying to troubleshoot a problem and need to do specific-level testing (e.g., to see if a student is having trouble with reading comprehension because he doesn't know how to tell relevant from irrelevant information); and
3. To monitor learning when a skill is being taught in isolation. (It is important to note that, even if an MM focuses on an isolated skill, it does not mean that skill should be taught in isolation. The skill is measured in isolation only for purposes of focus.)

The disadvantages of MMs come with their narrow focus. They are not good for surveying general levels of performance or for monitoring growth on long-term goals. Using a series of MMs to progress monitor will produce a profile of closely packed peaks and valleys that look like the teeth on a saw blade (see Figure 1.1). This profile emerges because,

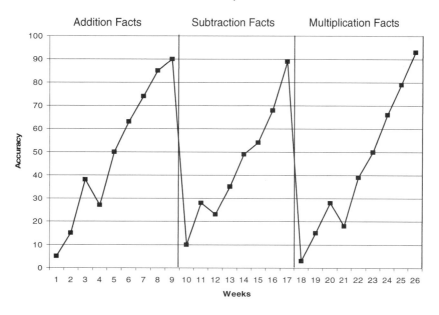

FIGURE 1.1. Example of an MM progress monitoring profile.

as soon as a student starts getting high scores on one of the very specific measures, a new one is introduced, and her score goes back down. That is called a *measurement shift* (or as we sometimes like to call it, "jumping off cliffs"). A GOM or SBM covering what amounts to the same slice of curriculum covered by a series of MMs won't produce these measurement shifts and will provide the long classic learning curve needed for decision making (see Figure 1.2).

A brief summary of the attributes for each type of measure is provided in Table 1.1.

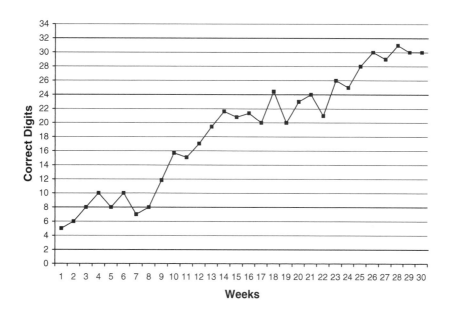

FIGURE 1.2. Example of a GOM or SBM progress monitoring profile.

TABLE 1.1. Comparison of the Three Types of Curriculum-Based Measures

General outcome measures (GOMs)	Skills-based measures (SBMs)	Mastery measures (MMs)
Primary uses		
• Screening • Survey-level testing • Progress monitoring	• Screening • Survey-level testing • Progress monitoring	• Diagnostic evaluation • Specific-level testing • To target content areas of concern • To target different proficiency levels and response types
Structure		
• Uses global/interactive tasks • Separate skills are not isolated or marked • Targets long-term goals • Often includes common classroom tasks	• Composed of mixed items drawn from a set of goals • Skills are usually sampled across a whole year's curriculum • Separate skills may be isolated or marked • Items are often cross-referenced to goals	• May only test one specific skill or short-term instructional objective • A large sample of performance is collected on each skill • Items are referenced to skills and/or proficiency levels • Some skills may be examined in isolation
Advantages		
• Provides perspective • Gives an overall impression of skill level • Useful for monitoring • No measurement shifts • Illustrates retention and generalization	• Gives an overall impression of skill level • Useful for monitoring • No measurement shifts • Illustrates retention	• Useful for double-checking a problem indicated on a GOM or SBM • Useful for checking hypotheses about missing skills or subskills • Provides focus
Disadvantages		
• Provides little diagnostic information • Doesn't provide information about specific skills • Often includes a high proportion of items that are either above or below the student's skill level • Some content areas don't have convenient capstone tasks	• Small sample for each goal limits diagnostic utility • Often includes a high proportion of items that are either above or below the student's skill level • May not require generalization or interactive use of the skill	• Doesn't provide the big picture (no generalization or application) • Skill–subskill relationships may not be real • Can't be used for progress monitoring

I HAVE NEVER SEEN CBM BEING USED— IF IT'S SO GREAT, WHY ISN'T IT MORE POPULAR?

There are probably several reasons. We think the main one is that, until recently, the general education community hasn't been asking the kinds of questions CBM answers, but that has changed. Part of the change is because of increased professional and legislative emphasis on accountability, and part of it is because of the popularity of the Dynamic Indicators of Basic Early Literacy Skills (DIBELS) and other CBM products. DIBELS started out as the application of CBM to early literacy skills, the same skills that were later given significance by the National Institute of Child Health and Human Development (2000) and National

Research Council (1998) reports. Within a couple of years after those reports came out, the DIBELS measures had been administered to literally millions of students in general education, particularly within the context of state-level reading improvement initiatives (e.g., Reading First programs).

There has been some debate about whether or not DIBELS is CBM. For the most part, it seems accurate to say that DIBELS applies CBM procedures to early reading tasks; however, there are differences in some scoring rules and item formats. Other modifications have also evolved with the development of web-based CBM management systems such as aimsweb, EasyCBM, and FastBridge Learning. Most of these changes seem to fall under the heading of fine-tuning and are probably to be expected as the application evolves for new populations and content areas.

Over the last decade more and more educators have become familiar with CBM. This is in large part due to the number of publishers who have CBM products available for the masses. It is also becoming more and more common for people to screen students on key skills like reading and math. Since curriculum-based measures offer some of the best psychometrically sound assessments for this purpose they are becoming more and more popular with educators in both the general and special education fields.

IS CBM USED WITH SPECIAL EDUCATION OR GENERAL EDUCATION?

CBM was originally used in special and remedial education because its ability to target specific skills and its sensitivity to instruction making it particularly useful for adjusting instruction to individual student needs, but special educators really aren't the only ones who do that. As mentioned, the use of CBM by general educators has been growing. This is, in part, due to the expansion of MTSS/RTI as a service delivery model. As also mentioned, everyone has become increasingly aware of the need to screen and progress monitor students in order to catch those who are falling behind as soon as possible. It is particularly important to progress monitor in high-impact content like reading, oral language, written expression, math, and social skills (as you'll find, not all of these areas are covered in this book). As a result, CBM is being increasingly adopted by whole school districts (and states) as a system for use with all students.

WHO GIVES CBM MEASURES?

It depends on why the measures are being given. Often curriculum-based measures are used three times over the course of the year to screen all students by looking at their level of performance and rate of progress in key skills like reading, math, and written expression. The reading comprehension, math, and written expression measures can all be group administered. If you are well prepared, math and written expression (depending on the grade level of the students) take from 5 to 10 minutes each. Oral reading requires individual administration and, if the flow of students and materials is managed smoothly, one person should be able to collect three individual reading samples from a student in another 5 minutes. The process takes, at most, 20 minutes of actual student testing time. Most of that time will be in group-administered activity. For the reading, because all students in a school are being tested during universal screening, the actual administration might be conducted by a team of general education teachers, special education teachers, school psychologists, reading specialists, and teaching assistants. We do not recommend using community contacts such as parents, volunteers, or peers for universal screening because of issues of confidentiality and organization.

Time spent preparing materials, organizing the space, and training people in how to administer, score, and record will pay off. Once all the testing is done, the data are then entered into a computer or web-based management system by someone on the school staff (again, not community volunteers). Many publishers also have the ability to directly enter student responses into a computer program, decreasing the time needed to manage the data and increasing the reliability of scoring since scores do not need to be transferred into another system. The other benefit of these computer programs is immediate assess to the data. In Chapter 11, we provide a guide for setting up and managing CBM measures and related activities.

Giving curriculum-based measures for the purpose of analyzing learning problems is a different matter. This book is really not about diagnostic assessment. Assessment for diagnostic purposes is usually carried out by someone who is an expert in the content area of concern as well as CBE. This person could be a general education teacher, special education teacher, content-area specialist, or school psychologist. When curriculum-based measures are given for analysis of a learning problem, there is no standard set of tests. Instead, specific measures are selected to check on the presence or absence of those skills suspected to be causing the problem. In order to do this, we need to have a set of these measures available, but unfortunately, there are not any such complete sets of measures. There are a few resources for developing or identifying such materials, and these are provided in the "Resources and/or Further Reading" section of Chapter 2.

Finally, CBM is also used to monitor the effectiveness of instruction by giving the students repeated measures of the same skills over time in order to see trends in their learning.

IF I WANT TO USE CBM, DOES THIS MEAN I'LL NEED TO MAKE TESTS OUT OF THE INSTRUCTIONAL MATERIALS I'M USING?

The short answer is "no." Because one of the hallmarks of CBM is technical adequacy, it is best to use published or otherwise openly available materials that have been evaluated. For universal screening and progress-monitoring decisions, reliable and valid instruments are a must. Enjoy having someone else do that work.

The long answer (in case you're wondering) is that this is an important question and an issue of some debate. The answer depends on the answer to another question that would seem to be fairly basic for people interested in CBM—namely, "What is the definition of *curriculum*?" We have said that curriculum is "what you teach," meaning it is the standards that must be met for students to achieve social and academic competence, but some people define curriculum to include "what you *use* to teach" (meaning the teaching materials being used).

If you take the "use" view, the curriculum is not just the skills that are taught, but also the approach through which they are being taught. Therefore, you would want program-specific measures (e.g., if your reading materials used numerous illustrations, you would have illustrations on your reading CBM).

If you take the "what" view of curriculum, you don't need to have tests using the same formats and examples as the instructional materials. You want tests that address the same skills and predict important outcome measures without using the exact same materials. You would be able to choose from already available generic measures. We subscribe to the "what" view. Here are some reasons for our position:

1. *Instructional programs don't follow the same sequences and schedules.* One of the biggest challenges in education is that what is taught and when it is taught really is not standardized across schools (even though the Common Core State Standards provide a fairly common set of standards to be achieved at the end of a grade level). It certainly is not standardized across published instructional programs. Obviously, this creates major problems in a mobile society.

2. *Program-specific tests may not tell you if the learning has generalized.* Our particular opinion is that you should carefully review and select the curriculum and then measure skills without being bound to any particular set of instructional materials. In fact, some may actually prefer to use CBM items that are somewhat different or at least mixed, to try to ensure that learning has generalized (you don't want a student who can only work problems that are presented in a certain format).

3. *Program-specific tests will make the teacher dependent on the program.* Instructional materials do not remain constant. They are often revised, or teachers select new ones. If teachers use program-specific tests, they will have to produce new ones every time a new program is selected. Wouldn't you rather put your energy into teaching?

WHERE DO I GET CBM MATERIALS?

There are many sources of CBM materials. Some must be purchased, and others are free. There are also materials that can be accessed on the web. Materials for the content areas addressed in this book will be referenced in those chapters. Just remember that when you select materials for CBM, you must have these two things:

1. *Alignment:* The materials must *match* the task, standards, and outcomes. This means the materials you select must sample the content you are interested in (e.g., reading) and call for the student to produce the same skills you are teaching (e.g., reading orally).
2. *Adequate sampling:* Be sure there are enough items and that the time interval is long enough to allow the student the opportunities needed to display her knowl-

edge. A good sample of behavior is necessary to make decisions about what a student knows.

Also remember that there is more to evaluation than giving a test. You have to score it properly, record the data accurately, and interpret them correctly. This book will give you information about CBM scoring rules and the interpretation of scores. Assessment is carried out to inform decision making; we need to know what the scores mean in order to use them.

SO, WHERE DO WE GO FROM HERE?

Our goal for this first chapter of the book has been to answer some of the fundamental questions that are asked about CBM in general terms of the "whats" and "whys." Chapter 2 provides additional detail putting CBM into a broader framework of decision making in education. For the rest of the book, we turn to the "hows," as in "How do I implement CBM?"

Chapters 3 through 9 each provide, for different areas of the curriculum, a rationale for using CBM, a list of materials needed and where to get those materials, directions and scoring procedures, how often it should be administered, how much time it will take to administer and score, information about the different types of CBM scores, how to write IEP goals and objectives, and frequently asked questions. Chapter 10 will take you through the process and procedures for setting goals and graphing the data as well as describe how CBM fits into an MTSS/RTI model. Chapter 11 provides a guide for how to use CBM, how to get it going, and how to sustain it. Appendix A provides norms for some of the reading CBM measures covered in Chapters 3 and 4, which have benchmarks that are provided within those chapters. All other norm tables are provided within the content chapters since there are no benchmarks currently available. Appendix B provides resources that can be photocopied and used while conducting CBM, including quick administration and scoring guides for each CBM skill covered in this book; two checklists for conducting CBM; and a graph to plot the data.

The chapters are structured this way to serve as a reference when you are implementing CBM. When using math materials, it is important to know about the administration directions, scoring, and standards for comparison that are specific to math. Graphing and setting or writing goals is a similar process no matter what the content area, so it wouldn't make sense to have to look up writing goals in the reading chapter when you want to write math goals!

CHAPTER 2

CBM for Assessment and Problem Solving

As educators we are active problem solvers. We constantly make decisions—the decisions that go into planning instruction and then the interactive decisions as those plans are adjusted, modified, and occasionally thrown out the window. The number of decisions made in an average school on any given day, given the mixture of age, content, and personalities found in classrooms, dwarfs the number made in any corporation (and we would argue that they are often more important). Making educational decisions is part of the work done in the context of a classroom, school, district, or state department of education, but the sorts of decisions made will be different depending on the work being done in these different contexts. One specific difference among these contexts is the balance of administrative work and teaching work.

The most administrative work occurs at the state department and school district levels. Administrators usually don't deliver instruction; they support and manage its delivery by providing leadership while advocating for, coordinating, and evaluating services. Teaching work pertains directly to teaching and learning. To do a good job at either administrative or teaching work, people need to solve problems and make good decisions. To carry out these tasks, at least four things are necessary:

1. A process for solving problems;
2. An understanding of the way decision making works in your job;
3. Good data; and
4. Adequate resources.

WHAT DO I NEED TO KNOW ABOUT EDUCATIONAL DECISION MAKING?

As much as we would like to, we really won't be covering everything you need to know about educational decision making in the next few pages. There are many different approaches to decision making, and CBM fits into many of them (a couple we recommend are listed in the "Resources and/or Further Reading" section). We will, however, cover the basics of how CBM fits within the framework of CBE (see Hosp, Hosp, Howell, & Allison, 2014, pp. 8–13, for more details).

The first thing to understand is that while you need good data to make good decisions, collecting good data doesn't guarantee anything. In other words:

- To make good decisions, you need to think productively.
- To think productively, you need good information.

so

- You must have good information to make good decisions!

Without good information (i.e., data) there won't be any good decisions (the "garbage in, garbage out" idea), but just collecting good information never helped anyone. You have to do something with the information. That is why, to understand CBM fully, you need to understand how it can be used to make decisions and solve problems.

The second thing to consider is that there are different kinds of decisions. Various models have been suggested for the classification of educational decisions. Within one of the most commonly used frameworks (and one that is not specific to reading), we design and implement evaluation around four specific program functions. This is accomplished by asking a question for each function and developing a measurement procedure and decision-making process to answer each question. The whole package includes:

Type 1: Universal Screening Decisions
- *Function:* To determine quickly if students are performing adequately and/or if they are at risk for future learning failure (and may need additional educational support).
- *Question:* "Which students are currently at risk for academic failure?"
- *Evaluation procedure:* An efficient procedure for assessing all students on key skills.
- *Note:* Because the need is to collect data that can be used to identify quickly students who are at risk, the results will only indicate the problem. They usually will not provide detailed guidance on how to correct it. Also, the term "at risk" is used to mean that the universal screening has predicted the student may not succeed without additional support. It does not imply that the student has some sort of disability or inherent limitation.

Type 2: Progress Monitoring Decisions
- *Function:* To ensure that instruction is working.
- *Question:* "Is the student making adequate progress toward important goals?"
- *Evaluation procedure:* A procedure is used that:
    1. Is directly aligned with what is being taught;
    2. Is sensitive to learning; and
    3. Can be given frequently.

- Ideally, this measure should also yield information that can be easily summarized and displayed on a chart or graph.
- *Note:* Progress monitoring may occur at the group level (as classes are screened/benchmarked three or four times a year) or for individual students. The frequency of monitoring should increase when a student is found to be experiencing a problem.

Type 3: Diagnostic Decisions

- *Function:* To develop an instructional plan in response to a significant problem.
- *Question:* "What and how should we teach this student?"
- *Evaluation procedure:* A personalized evaluation procedure that will allow the careful and systematic examination of a student's skills. This allows the selection of individual expectations and teaching approaches.
- *Note:* Diagnostic evaluation is reserved for those relatively rare instances when progress monitoring shows that various educational supports have not worked.

Type 4: Outcome Decisions

- *Function:* To determine and document the effectiveness of an educational program.
- *Question:* "Has this program been a success?"
- *Evaluation procedure:* A procedure is used that will supply the information needed to determine if program goals have been met.
- *Note:* Outcome decisions can be based on measures ranging from specific CBM reading passages to statewide high-stakes assessments. What tool you select depends largely on who you need to supply with the results.

CBM can contribute to making each of these four types of decisions. In this book, we focus primarily on how to do universal screening and progress monitoring. We will also mention when diagnostic evaluation may be needed and what kinds of tools you could use to carry it out.

The third thing to consider is the standard for comparison. With CBM, there are two standards that are commonly used: *benchmarks* and *norms*. A norm is basically the distribution of scores obtained by giving a measure to a randomly selected sample of students. Therefore, the scores in the norm represent the group from which the sample of students was selected. A *criterion* is a score that represents a desired level of performance. A benchmark is a specific type of criterion—the level of performance at or above which the student has a prespecified probability of demonstrating proficiency on an important outcome or standard (such as reading). Benchmarks and norms are both types of *standards* and should be established through a standardization process. This makes CBM no less *formal* than any other instrument used for accountability or eligibility.

There are some important differences between CBM and accountability/eligibility tests (AETs). Because AETs are designed to compare students to other students, it is necessary that when a group of students takes the test, its members get a range of scores. If everyone who took an AET got the same score—17, for example—there would be no way to say who was a high performer and who was a low performer; they would all just have 17. As a consequence, the primary purpose of accountability or eligibility, which is to allow the user to distinguish among students, would be lost. Therefore, the authors of AETs design their tests in ways that exaggerate the performance differences among students (i.e., promote variability in the scores). By doing so, they often decrease educators' ability to use the tests to make teaching decisions.

Here are some ways authors of AETs make sure students don't all get the same score:

How Authors Promote Variability on AETs	*The Effect This Can Have on Educational Value*
1. They put a range of items on the test, starting from very early skills and going to those that are advanced.	1. This produces a test that, for any student, has a large number of items that are either above or below his instructional level. As a result, much of his performance is on portions of the curriculum that are not currently relevant to his education. • CBM is aligned with instructional objectives, so it targets areas of current importance to the student.
2. They exclude items from the test that most students pass or that most students fail because these do not do a good job of discriminating among students.	2. Most students pass the items that most teachers find important and emphasize. This means that items covering important content may actually be thrown off an AET! • CBM, because it is curriculum-based, only includes items that match instructional goals.
3. Because the tests cover a wide range of difficulty, the authors can include only a few items for each skill (adding more items for each skill would make the test too long).	3. This means the sample of information collected for each skill is inadequate. • CBM provides enough items to collect an adequate sample of the student's performance.
4. Many AETs, particularly achievement measures, are designed to be group administered or machine scored. Therefore, they use identification response item formats (e.g., multiple choice).	4. This can cause misalignment between the conditions of testing and the behaviors teachers expect of students in the classroom. • CBM uses the same types of items students encounter in class and requires them to make the same sorts of responses.

It is probably obvious that we think curriculum-based measures are excellent tools for a variety of purposes; however (and this should be no surprise), advocates of other kinds of assessment tools would probably argue exactly the same thing. Therefore, the real question is "Which technology is the best for this purpose?" and that is a question usually followed by "As compared to what?"

Here are some attributes that any instructionally useful (that is our standard) measure/assessment should have. It should:

1. Be useful for *deciding "what" and/or "how" students need to be taught*;
2. Have *adequate reliability and validity* for the purposes used;
3. *Be standardized*, so we can judge the quality of a student's performance in relation to a target;
4. *Sample defined domains* of knowledge, content, and behavior so that we can tell what the student had to know and do to work the items;
5. Be *aligned with the curriculum* taught to the student;
6. *Collect an adequate sample* of behavior to allow us to draw conclusions with confidence;
7. *Use appropriate scoring rules* so that the results we get supply an accurate representation of the student's skills and knowledge;
8. Allow for the *collection of rate data* so that we can reach conclusions about the student's fluency as well as his accuracy; and
9. *Be easy to use* so it is efficient to administer and score (and all instruction in the school doesn't have to be shut down for 2 weeks).

Every measure that we use does not need to have every one of these attributes as long as they are all covered within our total assessment package, but it really would be better if they all did because each of these nine attributes is important to instructional utility.

ARE CURRICULUM-BASED MEASURES STANDARDIZED TESTS?

The term *standardized* has two meanings: The first is that the test is given in a standard fashion, meaning that there are administration and scoring procedures set out for everyone to follow; the second is that a *standard* (the benchmark or norm) has been established so scores can be interpreted in terms of a validated referent. The process of developing the standard that will be used for these comparisons is called standardization.

CBM meets both of these definitions of standardized. It comes with administration and scoring procedures that need to be followed (and will be provided in this text) and with standards, in the form of performance criteria or norms that can be used to allow interpretation. These will also be provided when available.

Most curriculum-based measures are criterion referenced. The criteria are the same ones found in curriculum standards or objectives. They have nothing to do with how well other students may or may not be performing. For example, if a student is in the fall of his fifth-grade year, he should read aloud from fifth-grade material at about 111 words correctly per minute with 97% accuracy or better. That criterion for oral reading specifies a desired level of performance even if most students in the class are reading 65 words or fewer correctly per minute.

HOW RELIABLE AND VALID IS CBM?

We're glad you asked!

While some measures are more reliable or valid than others, all the measures presented in this book meet general standards for reliability and validity. There have been more than 100 studies on the reliability or validity of CBM, and these have been summarized and synthesized into other articles and chapters. You can find references to some of these in the "Resources and/or Further Reading" at the end of this chapter and in the References at the end of the book.

There are some CBM measures that aren't presented in this book, but that doesn't mean that they aren't reliable or valid—it means we didn't have room for them or the research is still in its infancy. Since new CBMs are still under development in several areas, it's important that you as the consumer check out their reliability and validity to make sure they're appropriate for you to use.

WHERE DO THEY GET THE PERFORMANCE STANDARDS USED IN CBM?

The most common way that CBM performance standards are set can be called a *predictive validity* model. This involves empirically or statistically determining the level of performance that reliably predicts successful performance on a different outcome measure, usually at a future date. For example, we might want to know how many words read correctly to expect at the beginning of second grade to predict who will earn a proficient score on the state's second-grade accountability test (given at the end of the year). When performance standards are set this way, you should consider what is being predicted and if it is a skill or performance level one actually wants students to work toward and meet.

This type of performance standard is generally referred to as a *benchmark*. Here, the term indicates a score and is used as a noun, while previously the term *benchmarking* has been used to indicate collecting data for the purpose of universal screening (we use the term *universal screening* rather than *benchmarking* to avoid confusion). Benchmarks are scores that have been determined to predict later success on related tasks. Therefore, they are appropriate criteria to use for current performance. The benchmark score, however, is not the highest score, or even the middle score, but rather the lowest score one would accept that would indicate a student is *not* at risk for future academic failure. Even if students were not performing at an acceptable level at the beginning of the year (when the class was screened), as long as they make progress that will take them to mastery by the end of the year, we can feel confident that they will be performing proficiently and will not be at risk for later academic difficulty. Similar to taking a driver's test, everyone who gets a driver's license has to perform at or above a certain criterion level on the test. It doesn't matter how other people your age scored on the test—which is the basis for the other method of setting performance standards.

Another common way to set performance standards is to use *norm sampling*. This involves testing all students at the end of the school year (or three times during the year) and using the average scores at a grade level or some percentage of them as the target level of performance for that grade from then on. Before the widespread development and use of benchmarks, educators relied on norms to help them determine expectations related to how well a student scored. Valid representative national norms have been assembled on some curriculum-based measures (particularly in the area of reading). Many school districts prefer to use local norms. The obvious danger with local norms is that, in some schools, the average level of performance may be inadequate. In this case (and others) local norms might give a false impression of student proficiency.

While we struggle to find a use for norms, we also understand they have a long tradition in using CBM data. For this reason, we are providing normative data for those CBM tasks for which they are available. We have supplied norms within the content chapters for those CBM measures that do not yet have benchmarks that are empirically established. Appendix A provides norms for those curriculum-based measures that do have benchmarks, including Early Reading CBM, Oral Passage Reading CBM, and Maze CBM.

HOW CAN CBM BE USED FOR UNIVERSAL SCREENING?

Universal screening is typically carried out using GOMs or SBMs. It is applied to find students who are falling behind or who are at risk for academic failure. An ideal universal screening test is quick and easy to give. It doesn't need to provide much information. It only needs to be a good predictor of future success (or failure) in the content area it covers. If universal screening signals a problem or potential problem, the student is typically supplied with educational support and increased progress monitoring. In cases where the problem seems to be extreme, it may be decided that the student needs to be given a diagnostic evaluation immediately. Often, students who have this level of need will already be known. Diagnostic evaluation is usually reserved for these students and those who, according to progress monitoring, fail to respond to instruction.

It is recommended all students be screened at least three times a year in order to examine if a student is on track for being proficient by the end of the school year. In essence it allows us to ask "Is this student *at risk* for academic failure by the end of the year?" Universal screening produces a score to be compared to a benchmark and typically occurs two or three times per year, in the fall, winter, and spring.

This is done in the way that vital signs (temperature, heart rate, blood pressure) might be quickly checked by a physician or nurse. This analogy, that CBM can be used to check certain key skills indicating a student's "academic health," has been popularized by Mark Shinn (1989). It is based on the idea that performance on some tasks, while not giving the information one would need to plan an intervention, can be used to indicate the strength of a student's skill within a curriculum domain. If the score is outside of the acceptable range, professionals are alerted to the existence of a problem requiring additional attention. Using

CBM in this fashion is particularly appropriate because of its efficiency, sensitivity to learning, and direct relationship to learning outcomes.

Universal screening three times a year also provides data to ask additional questions like "Is our core instruction meeting the needs of most of our students?" and "Are all subgroups being successful?" If core instruction were sufficient you would expect to see around 80% of students at or above the benchmark for each testing period. This 80% means students receiving only core instruction and not students who are also receiving interventions. You would expect the same trends to be consistent across subgroups as they occur across the entire school population.

CBM can be used to find two indicators of a problem: first, low *performance* (or level of performance) in a key skill area; and second, low *progress* (or rate of progress) in the acquisition of key skills. By *acquisition* we mean learning, as seen in changes of student performance over time. As long as sufficiently sensitive tools are used for universal screening, the presence or absence of these changes can be seen. This means universal screening should be repeated for all students several times a year, usually a minimum of three. After a student has taken the universal screening measures, his scores are compared to both level of performance and rate of progress expectations to make universal screening decisions. In this system, it is actually possible to recognize a learning problem in a student who performs relatively well on the tests but is not making progress. Here is what this might look like: A student named Larry moves into a new school district and on the fall oral reading universal screening gets a fairly high score. When tested again, in the winter universal screening, Larry gets the same score. This means he has not made progress. While he is still a high performer relative to many of his peers, his peers have made progress; they are currently low performers making good progress, while he, at the winter universal screening, is a relatively high performer making no progress. Given this information, you would worry more about Larry than about the other students.

CBM allows us to examine learning in the form of progress data. We can collect the progress data because CBM is a direct measure of what is taught and can be used in a repeated measurement format. Other commonly used measures can't be employed this way. Again, oral passage reading (which is a GOM for reading) is a good example of a universal screening task as it is quick (three 1-minute sessions per student) and reflects the integration of many separate reading skills. Therefore, three 1-minute timed oral readings can make an excellent screener for reading problems.

Special considerations for universal screening include testing at the appropriate time. For example, we do not recommend universally screening students during the first 2 weeks of school for two reasons: Students often need instruction to recapture some skills they may have forgotten, and not all students may have enrolled or started to attend school. This means early universal screening may miss some students who need help. Also, teachers may be reassigned based on final enrollment figures.

Universal screening too early might cause you to overidentify students who appear to need additional instructional help. This can affect the use of resources and take valuable time and instruction away from those students who need it most. Therefore, we recommend waiting at least 2 weeks after the start of school to screen all students and avoiding winter and spring universal screening dates that occur right after long breaks.

Universal Screening Summary

- *Evaluation question:* "Which students are at risk for academic failure?"
- *Function:* Universal screening procedures are used to check all students in order to identify those needing extra help or alternate forms of instruction.
- *Procedure:* Check "vital signs." Use CBM data to sort students quickly according to their level of performance and rate of progress. Choose their current program, a new program, or additional diagnostic evaluation according to their needs.

HOW CAN CBM BE USED FOR PROGRESS MONITORING?

Our knowledge of educational programming has not evolved to the point where we can guarantee positive results from every teaching decision made (incidentally, neither has the knowledge level in psychology, law, medicine, finance, or government). Therefore, we need to monitor the effects of decisions and instruction to see if they are working. Consistent monitoring of student learning coupled with a set of formal instructional decision rules can greatly improve the effectiveness of instruction. In fact, it is one of the most powerful innovations that can be introduced in a classroom or school system.

We use progress monitoring to inform the decisions we make during the process of instruction or intervention. This is true at any program level. Progress monitoring can inform adjustments in statewide literacy initiatives or the multiplication instruction of a single student; the principles are the same. To succeed, the progress-monitoring tool must be sensitive to the impact of the instruction being delivered. Translated into educational practice, this means educators need to monitor with a measure that responds to the small changes in behavior resulting from day-to-day learning. That is the only way to get the feedback needed to make timely adjustments in instruction. The monitoring tools used for instructional interventions must:

- Directly sample what is being taught;
- Get an adequate sample of behavior; and
- Allow for repeated administration.

While most curriculum-based measures conform to these criteria, we often switch back to the GOMs or SBMs used for universal screening when we monitor progress. This is because the purpose of our intervention is to improve the student's skills to the point that she would not have failed the original universal screening (and would never have been identified as someone needing support). In addition, GOMs and SBMs have the advantage of adding the broader perspective of complex tasks. For example, writing samples may be used to collect monitoring data for written expression because they reflect a cluster of related skills even though a student's instruction may only be focusing on one or two specific skills within that cluster. (Similarly, it is common to use reading passages from the student's grade level to monitor her reading acquisition. In this way you can see how she is advancing toward proficiency in the material with which she is expected to work.)

Last, it is important to note again that the sensitivity of a progress monitoring system does not depend entirely on the way the CBM measure functions each time it is given. It also depends on whether or not the measure can be given multiple times. As a general rule, the more frequently you measure (typically one or two times per week for CBM), the more sensitive your data set will be to the influence of your intervention and, of course, the more frequently you will be able to make data-based decisions about the quality of your program. CBM is designed for this sort of frequent use, whereas other types of measures can't be repeated without jeopardizing their validity. One reason CBM works this way is that, as you may recall from Chapter 1, it was originally designed specifically for progress monitoring.

Using the universal screening data, we can identify which students' progress should be monitored. The purpose of progress monitoring is to ensure students are benefiting from the instruction they are receiving. This is accomplished by frequently checking their progress toward an end-of-year benchmark score. Progress monitoring is recommended for those students who are at risk for academic failure. This can be conceptualized in most cases as those not meeting the benchmark score during the universal screening windows. This group will often include students with disabilities as well as students who are merely behind their same-grade peers. Because these students are already behind, it is critical to monitor their progress often and consistently. By "often," we mean at least once per week. By "consistently," we mean using CBM assessments that are at the same difficulty level. If the criterion changes from week to week, we cannot determine if the student is making adequate progress given the instruction she is receiving or if the change in scores reflects a change in assessment. Producing multiple versions of passages that are of equivalent difficulty can be very difficult and time consuming. This is why we recommend purchasing commercial materials to reduce variability.

Progress monitoring weekly allows us to ask questions like "Is this student benefiting from the instruction she is receiving?" and "Is this intervention helping the majority of students who have received it?" For an individual, it provides that database needed to determine if instructional changes need to be made or if the student is progressing at a rate that will allow him or her to hit the end-of-year benchmark by the end of the year. If students can reach that benchmark, it would indicate they are on track and *not* at risk. In addition, for all students who have received the intervention you now have a larger database to compare their progress and determine if the intervention is effective in general. This can be accomplished by taking an average of the slopes for every student who received the intervention and by counting the percentage of other students who also hit the end-of-year benchmark score. Those interventions that had the largest growth *and* have the largest percentage of students who reached the end-of-year benchmark would be the ones to keep using. Those interventions that did not show much growth or where no students reached the end-of-year benchmark should be eliminated. At the end of each school year, all interventions can be reviewed using these two criteria and plans can be made for the following year. If *no* interventions are looking promising based on the progress-monitoring data, this might have more to do with the implementation fidelity and less to do with the overall intervention.

Special considerations for progress-monitoring data include not letting the student take home the progress-monitoring material to practice. It is important to separate testing from teaching. If you want a student to have more practice on the skill that is similar to the test, then it should be something that is embedded in student materials and not testing materials. For example, if you are assessing sight words, you should use your own bank of words from the curriculum or a high-frequency word list to send home and *not* the words directly on the CBM assessment.

Progress Monitoring Summary

- *Evaluation questions:* "Is the intervention working?" and "What changes should we make?"
- *Function:* To ensure that instruction is working; to signal when a change is needed and to guide adjustments in the program.
- *Procedure:* Use measures that reflect responses to instructional interventions or programs in terms of progress toward the acquisition of skills and meeting of standards.

As already explained, it is more important to see that students are progressing adequately through the curriculum than it is to require them to learn from any particular method. This leads to another basic principle of progress monitoring in education: There is no reason to monitor if we don't intend to make changes. If a student (or group) is not progressing adequately, it is the teacher's (or organization's) responsibility to try to find a new approach to the instruction of that skill. While universal screening and progress-monitoring measures may alert you to the need for a change, they will not always give you the information you need to decide what kind of change you should make.

When progress monitoring indicates that the student is learning, the logical thing to do is to stay with the current program. If the indications are that the student is not learning, this can signal the need for a diagnostic evaluation. Diagnostic evaluation is not the focus of this text (it is covered in detail in a problem-solving process such as CBE and is the focus of *The ABCs of Curriculum-Based Evaluation*; see the "Resources and/or Further Reading" section of this chapter).

One of the most likely explanations for a student's failure to perform a task is that he is missing the necessary prior knowledge to succeed. To put it another way, the most likely reason a student can't do something is that he doesn't know how. Therefore, when targeting inquiry and measurement, the most important learner characteristic to examine is the student's prior knowledge. For example, if a student is having trouble reading his sixth-grade history text, you would target the skills needed to read that book. These skills should reside in the curriculum.

When conducting a diagnostic curriculum-based evaluation, you don't want to let your thinking stray from the prior knowledge hypothesis. If you do, you may end up targeting and testing things like learning aptitude, intelligence, cognitive processing characteristics, perceptual abilities, auditory discrimination, visual–motor integration, or even general achievement. These are not examples of the skills and knowledge that make up the curriculum. Most of them are constructs that have only a hypothetical and/or correlational relationship to the curriculum. Instead, tools such as the Multilevel Academic Skills Inventory (MASI) can help maintain the focus on prior knowledge. They can also help pinpoint what specific skills need to be taught in a logical scope and sequence.

In order to target measurement and problem solving in a curriculum-based paradigm, you need an understanding of the curriculum area and direct measures of the student's skills. This means that, while your knowledge of the curriculum will help you come up with the targets, you will need CBM to check the student's status and find out if he doesn't know the key prerequisite skills. This is why selection of a correct standard and analysis of existing knowledge is so important.

In a well-designed curriculum, essential prerequisite knowledge is located at lower levels in the skill sequences. When you conduct the inquiry, CBM is the best way to get a good handle on how well the student has mastered those prerequisites. The GOMs and SBMs used for universal screening often do not supply enough of a sample or the specific focus you need to allow this sort of analysis. Therefore, specific-level MMs designed to target particular skills are commonly used for the diagnostic function.

HOW DO I USE THE INFORMATION TO WRITE INDIVIDUALIZED EDUCATION PLAN GOALS AND OBJECTIVES?

CBM data are an excellent source for writing individualized education plan (IEP) goals and objectives. Because educators can monitor how well the student is doing on a weekly basis, they no longer have to hold their breath and hope that when they test her at the end of the year she will have reached her goal(s). CBM is the best measurement system currently available to monitor students' progress toward long-term goals. The best part about using CBM to monitor progress is that it is sensitive to student improvement so that if the student is learning the material, you will see an increase in her CBM score each week. The reverse also holds true: If the student is not learning the material, you will not see an improvement each week. This allows teachers to make instructional changes as often as needed. Using CBM in this way stacks the cards in the student's favor to reach the goal and objectives the team has developed.

In addition, CBM is extremely efficient to use for writing goals and objectives because it provides a way to clearly define and observe the behaviors we are most interested in. For reading, these behaviors are saying letter sounds, reading words, and reading passages. Correctly restoring missing words is the behavior for comprehension. Therefore, incorporating CBM information into writing goals and objectives provides clear and straightforward criteria on which one can gauge students' success. To write a good goal and objective you will need to include the following seven components:

1. *Time* (the amount of time the goal is written for, typically 1 year)
   "In 1 year . . ."
2. *Learner* (the student for whom the goal is being written)
   " . . . Jose will . . ."
3. *Behavior* (the specific skill the student will demonstrate)
   " . . . read aloud . . ."

4. *Level* (the grade the content is from)
   " . . . second-grade . . . "
5. *Content* (what the student is learning about)
   " . . . reading . . . "
6. *Material* (what the student is using)
   " . . . passage from oral passage reading CBM progress monitoring material . . . "
7. *Criteria* (the expected level of performance, including time and accuracy)
   "90 words correctly in 1 minute with greater than 95% accuracy."

Procedures for setting criteria are provided in Chapter 10.

Additional online resources on CBM are listed in the "Resources and/or Further Reading" section at the end of the chapter. Additional information for specific curriculum-based measures will be shared in Chapters 3–9, which cover individual content areas.

RESOURCES AND/OR FURTHER READING

Big Ideas in Beginning Reading (*reading.uoregon.edu*). Includes information related to the research, assessments, and instruction for phonemic awareness, alphabetic principle, accuracy and fluency with text, vocabulary, and comprehension.

Hosp, J. L., Hosp, M. K., Howell, K. W., & Allison, R. (2014). *The ABCs of curriculum-based evaluation: A practical guide to effective decision making.* New York: Guilford Press.

Intervention Central—CBM Warehouse (*www.interventioncentral.org/curriculum-based-measurement-reading-math-assesment-tests*). Includes CBM materials for screening and progress monitoring along with information on using CBM and interpreting results from CBM data.

National Center on Intensive Intervention (*www.intensiveintervention.org*). Includes charts evaluating CBM tools for progress monitoring in academics and behavior along with webinars, and other publications related to assessment and interventions.

National Center on Response to Intervention (*www.rti4success.org*). Includes a chart evaluating CBM tools for screening along with webinars, training modules, and other publications related to RTI.

National Center on Student Progress Monitoring (*www.studentprogress.org*). Includes CBM articles, PowerPoints, presentations, and other resources about CBM measures and using CBM data.

Research Institute on Progress Monitoring (*www.progressmonitoring.org*). Includes CBM reports and materials for Early Numeracy, Significant Cognitive Disabilities, and Early Writing.

Shapiro, E. S. (2010). *Academic skills problems: Direct assessment and intervention* (4th ed.). New York: Guilford Press.

Special Connections, University of Kansas (*www.specialconnections.ku.edu*). Includes CBM articles, case studies, and others resources on data-based decision making and behavior plans.

CHAPTER 3

How to Conduct Early Reading CBM

WHY SHOULD I CONDUCT EARLY READING CBM?

The earlier you detect whether a student is on track to be a successful reader the better your chances are of intervening early and changing the trajectory of that student's reading skills. Advancements in Early Reading CBM, particularly in kindergarten and first grade, have allowed us to expand the number of measures to share. While there are over 30 years of research supporting the use of CBM in reading and math, Early Reading CBM has only taken off in the past 10 years. Just as traditional curriculum-based measures have always included rate and accuracy, most Early Reading measures share these same features. It is critical to understand that rate, often referred to as fluency, allows us to determine how automatically students can perform a task. Automaticity is important because it demonstrates the student has mastered the skill. Rate also explains significant unique variance in reading ability, making it more useful than traditional measures that rely on accuracy alone (Fuchs, Fuchs, Hosp, & Jenkins, 2001).

Early Reading CBM is also necessary within any good MTSS/RTI framework. This is because early identification is one of the most critical components, and Early Reading CBM allows you to screen all students three times a year. Students who have mastered certain early reading skills (e.g., naming pictures and letters, segmenting and blending sounds in words, identifying letter sounds, reading basic words) in kindergarten and first grade are much more likely to continue on the road to becoming successful readers. Those students who have not mastered these early reading skills by kindergarten and first grade are at risk of continuing to fall further and further behind their peers and not becoming good readers. The research on early intervention tells us that the chance of helping students become proficient readers is greatly increased the earlier one intervenes (Snow, Burns, & Griffin, 1998; Vellutino et al., 2006). Waiting until second or third grade stacks the deck against students, making it much more difficult to help these students become proficient readers. The good news is that we know we can teach these important early reading skills and change the trajectory of these students' achievement in reading.

Using Early Reading CBM is essential in determining who is at risk early on so that intervention and progress monitoring can start right away. Once students are identified as being at risk, we also need to monitor their progress using Early Reading CBM as a way to identify which students are not making adequate progress given the instruction they are receiving so that appropriate instructional changes can be made. One of the unique features of CBM is that many of the assessments that are used to identify which students are at risk (i.e., universal screening) are also used to monitor their progress (i.e., progress monitoring), making it very efficient with regard to cost and time needed to implement. The progress-monitoring data provide a database for each student so that instructional decisions can be made in a timely manner. These measures require the student to be accurate as well as fluent, allowing one to determine how automatic students are at performing a task. Remember, automaticity is important because it represents a higher level of skill mastery.

Early Reading CBM consists of many tasks, such as rhyming, sound identification, concepts of print, onset sounds, word segmenting, word blending, letter naming, letter sounds, nonsense words, word identification, and sentence reading. These tasks cover many different aspects of literacy skills that have been shown to be predictive of later reading success. Table 3.1 shows a comparison of four commonly used commercial products and the early literacy skills addressed by each. This is not an exhaustive list of publishers but rather a representative sample. We will provide detailed information for those skills that are identified by at least two of the four publishers, and a brief overview for those identified by only one publisher.

TABLE 3.1. Common Commercial CBM Products by Early Literacy Skill

Early literacy skill assessed	aimsweb	DIBELS	Easy CBM	FastBridge Learning
Concepts of print				Concepts of Print
Rhyming				Word Rhyming
Blending				Word Blending
Segmenting	Phoneme Segmentation	Phoneme Segmentation Fluency	Phoneme Segmenting	Word Segmenting
Onset sounds		First Sound Fluency		Onset Sounds
Letter names	Letter Naming	Letter Naming Fluency	Letter Names	Letter Names
Letter sounds	Letter Sound		Letter Sounds	Letter Sounds
Nonsense words	Nonsense Word	Nonsense Word Fluency		Nonsense Word Reading
Decodable words				Decodable Word Reading
Sight words			Word Reading Fluency	Sight Word Reading
Sentence reading				Sentence Reading

First, we provide a brief description of those additional skills that are only available from a single publisher. This provides a more comprehensive view of all of the possible Early Reading curriculum-based measures. Next, we provide a detailed description of those skills that are common across publishers and share what materials are needed along with the administration and scoring rules.

OVERVIEW OF EARLY READING CURRICULUM-BASED MEASURES IDENTIFIED BY ONE PUBLISHER

Concepts of Print CBM

Concepts of print is a task designed to assess students' understanding of the structures related to books and text on a page. The student is shown a piece of paper with items or words on it. The teacher/examiner asks 12 questions related to the items in front of the student (e.g., "Point to where I should start reading the sentence"). To be marked correct, the student must point to the correct items or spot on the paper. This task is timed on how long it takes (in seconds) to respond to a total of 12 questions, producing an accuracy and rate score for the number of correctly answered questions.

Rhyming CBM

Rhyming is a task designed to assess phonological awareness. The student is shown a page with a set of pictures. The teacher/examiner says a word and asks the student to point to the picture that rhymes or to provide a new word that rhymes. To be marked correct, the student must point to the correct picture or say a correct rhyming word. This task is timed on how long it takes (in seconds) to respond to a total of 16 items, producing an accuracy and rate score for the number of correctly answered items.

Word Blending CBM

Word blending is a task designed to assess phonemic awareness. The teacher/examiner reads aloud a list of three- or four-phoneme words by sounds and the student must take the individual sounds and produce the whole word. To be marked correct, the student must say the correct word from the sounds provided. This task is timed on how long it takes (in seconds) to respond to a total of 10 words, producing an accuracy and rate score for the number of correctly answered items.

Decodable Words CBM

Decodable words is a task designed to assess the reading of phonetically regular words. The student is shown a page of 50 three-letter words (consonant–vowel–consonant). The teacher/examiner asks the student to read each word allowed. To be marked correct, the student must say the correct sounds and/or word. This task is timed for 1 minute, producing an accuracy and rate score for the number of correctly produced letter sounds and the number of whole words read.

Sentence Reading CBM

Sentence reading is a task designed to assess oral passage reading using a modified format. Instead of the entire passage being presented on a page, the passage is broken down into sentences and pictures across several pages. The student is shown a page with sentence(s) and a picture. The teacher/examiner asks the student to read each sentence aloud. To be marked correct, the student must read each word in the correct order as it appears on the page. This task is timed for 1 minute, producing an accuracy and rate score for the number of words read correctly.

In the following sections, we provide detailed descriptions of six Early Reading CBM skills that are common across publishers and share what materials are needed, along with the administration and scoring rules. To help you easily find materials, we provide sources of common commercial Early Reading CBM products in Box 3.1.

ONSET SOUNDS CBM

Onset Sounds CBM is designed to assess phonological awareness and specifically the ability to produce the beginning sounds in words and/or to respond to beginning sounds by pointing to pictures that represent initial sounds in words.

Materials Needed to Conduct Onset Sounds CBM

1. Different but equivalent stimuli sheets (student and/or teacher/examiner copies).
2. Directions for administering and scoring Onset Sounds CBM.
3. A writing utensil and clipboard or computer to enter student responses.
4. A stopwatch or countdown timer that displays seconds.
5. A quiet testing environment to work with students.
6. An equal-interval graph or a graphing program to plot the data.

Onset Sounds CBM Sheets

Onset Sounds CBM sheets should have different items. Some publishers assess this skill entirely auditorily by producing sounds (e.g., DIBELS, First Sound Fluency), while others use a combination of pointing to pictures that represent sounds and producing sounds (e.g., FastBridge Learning, Onset Sounds). For the purposes of discussing the directions, scoring, and additional considerations we will be referring to the FastBridge Learning materials. We recommend people look at the specific measures they will be using to ensure they follow the administration and scoring rules applicable for that specific measure, as there are variations among publishers.

BOX 3.1. Where to Find Premade Early Reading CBM Materials

$ indicates there is a cost for the sheets or lists and/or graphing program.
⌨ indicates computerized administration available.
✍ indicates data management and graphing available.
S indicates Spanish measures are available.

aimsweb (Pearson) $⌨✍S

Website: *www.aimsweb.com*

Phone: 866-313-6194

Products: • Letter Naming   • Phoneme Segmentation
            • Letter Sound   • Nonsense Word

Dynamic Indicators of Basic Early Literacy Skills (DIBELS) ✍S

Website: *dibels.org*

Phone: 888-943-1240

Products: • First Sound Fluency   • Phoneme Segmentation Fluency
            • Letter Naming Fluency   • Nonsense Word Fluency

EasyCBM $✍

Website: *easycbm.com*

Phone: 800-323-9540

Products: • Letter Names   • Phoneme Segmenting
            • Letter Sounds   • Word Reading Fluency

Edcheckup $✍

Website: *www.edcheckup.com*

Phone: 612-454-0074

Products: • Letter Sounds
            • Isolated Words

FastBridge Learning $⌨✍S

Website: *fastbridge.org*

Phone: 612-424-3714

Products: • Concepts of Print   • Word Segmenting
            • Onset Sounds   • Sight Word Reading
            • Letter Names   • Decodable Word Reading
            • Letter Sounds   • Nonsense Word Reading
            • Word Rhyming   • Sentence Reading
            • Word Blending   • Oral Language (Sentence Repetition)

Intervention Central ✍S

Website: *www.interventioncentral.org*

Products: • Letter Name Fluency   • Dolch Word List Fluency
            • Letter Sound Fluency

(continued)

Project AIM (Alternative Identification Models) ✍

Website: *www.glue.umd.edu/%7Edlspeece/cbmreading/index.html*

Phone: 301-405-6514

Products: • Letter Sound Test

System to Enhance Educational Performance (STEEP) $✍

Website: *www.isteep.com*

Phone: 800-881-9142

Products: • Letter Sounds

Vanderbilt University $ (copying, postage, and handling only)

Website: *www.peerassistedlearningstrategies.com*

Phone: 615-343-4782

E-mail: *lynn.a.davies@vanderbilt.edu*

Products: • Letter Sound Fluency
            • Word Identification Fluency

We recommend administering all universal screening assessments in one testing session to save setup time and for consistency in obtaining an accurate score, but they can occur across consecutive days if needed. If three samples of the same CBM task are to be administered, then the median score is used for the final score and can also be placed as the first data point on the student's graph. After that, 20–30 different but equivalent sheets will be used to monitor student progress in reading throughout the year.

Onset Sounds CBM must be administered individually. Two copies of the sheet will be needed. The student should have a copy of the Onset Sounds CBM sheet in front of him, and the teacher/examiner should either have a copy of the Onset Sounds CBM sheet in front of her on the computer screen or a paper copy to write on and a writing utensil, as well as a timer and the directions. See Figures 3.1 and 3.2 for examples of each type of sheet.

Directions and Scoring Procedures for Onset Sounds CBM

For your convenience, Appendix B includes a reproducible version of the directions and scoring rules for Onset Sounds CBM.

Directions for Onset Sounds CBM[1]

1. Place the Onset Sounds CBM practice copy with the four pictures in front of the student. There are five pages total (one practice, four test pages). Place the remaining test pages face down beside the teacher/examiner.
2. Place the teacher/examiner copy on the clipboard or pull up the scoring sheet on the computer screen so the student cannot see it.

---

[1]Adapted with permission from FastBridge Learning.

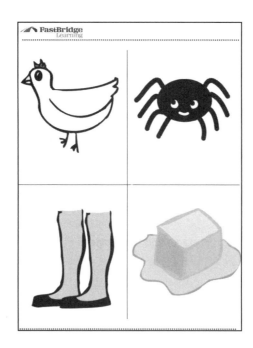

FIGURE 3.1. Example of student Onset Sounds CBM sheet. Reprinted with permission from FastBridge Learning.

FastBridge
Learning

<u>Scoring Sheet - Onset Sounds</u>

ITEM	QUESTIONS	CORRECT ANSWERS	
Read ► This is a chicken, spider, legs, and ice.			
1.	Which one begins with /sp/?	0	1
2.	Which one begins with /l/?	0	1
3.	Which one begins with /ch/?	0	1
4.	What's the first sound in the word "ice"? (point to ice)	0	1
Read ► This is a monkey, grass, ambulance, and road.			
5.	Which one begins with /a/?	0	1
6.	Which one begins with /m/?	0	1
7.	Which one begins with /g/?	0	1
8.	What's the first sound in the word "road"? (point to road)	0	1
Read ► This is a pizza, table, flower, and nail.			
9.	Which one begins with /fl/?	0	1
10.	Which one begins with /n/?	0	1
11.	Which one begins with /t/?	0	1
12.	What's the first sound in the word "pizza"? (point to pizza)	0	1
Read ► This is juice, broom, thermometer, and hand.			
13.	Which one begins with /b/?	0	1
14.	Which one begins with /h/?	0	1
15.	Which one begins with /th/?	0	1
16.	What's the first sound in the word "juice?" (point to juice)	0	1

Total Seconds (optional)__________ Total Items Correct______

FIGURE 3.2. Example of teacher/examiner Onset Sounds CBM sheet. Reprinted with permission from FastBridge Learning.

3. Say: *"We will do an activity with word sounds. Look at these pictures. This is a key, bat, dolphin, and water* (point to each picture as you say the word)*. Which one of these words begins with the /k/ sound—'key,' 'bat,' 'dolphin,' or 'water'?"*
   a. If correct, say: *"Good. 'Key' begins with /k/"* and move to practice item 2.
   b. If incorrect, say: *"Let's try again. 'Key'* (point to the key) *begins with /k/. /k/—'key.'* (Remove your finger from the picture.) *Which one of these words begins with /k/?"*
   c. If correct, say: *"Good, 'key' begins with /k/"* (point to the key).
   d. If incorrect, say: *"'Key' begins with /k/"* (point to the key) and move to extra practice 1.
4. For practice item 2, say: *"Let's try something different. This time, I'll say the word and then you give the first sound.* (Point to the bat.) *'Bat.' The first sound in the word 'bat' is /b/. Now you try. What is the first sound in the word 'water'?"* (Point to the picture of water.)
   a. If correct, say: *"Good. 'Water' begins with /w/"* and move to begin test.
   b. If incorrect, say: *"Let's try again. 'Water'* (point to the water) *begins with /w/. /w/— 'water.' What is the first sound in the word 'water'?* (point to the water). *Remember, just tell the sound."*
   c. If correct, say: *"Good, 'water' begins with /w/."*
   d. If incorrect, say: *"Listen, 'water' begins with /w/. The first sound is /w/"* and begin test.
5. To begin test, say: *"I will show you more pictures. Remember to listen to the names of the pictures and answer each question. Let's begin."* (Start timer.)
6. Place the first Onset Sounds CBM test sheet with the four pictures in front of the student. Ask each question clearly and point to each picture as you say the word. Once a student responds, ask the next question immediately. Do not give any more feedback about the student's response. If the student pauses for 5 seconds without responding to an item, count the item incorrect and continue with the next item. Continue through item 16 using prompts provided on the FastBridge Learning assessment page.
7. Stop timer after item 16 is completed or if test is discontinued.

Scoring Onset Sounds CBM

Submit the results using the online system. Or:

1. Count the total number of correct items (out of 16) and note how many seconds it took to complete.
2. Calculate rate: (Total number correct ÷ total seconds to complete) × 60 = rate score per minute.
3. Calculate accuracy: Total correct ÷ total items attempted = percent correct.

SCORED AS CORRECT

Onset Sounds CBM is scored based on the correct production or identification of the initial sound(s). Each correct initial sound is marked as correct (1) on the score sheet.

- Pronounced correctly: The first sound or sounds are pronounced correctly.
  - *Example:* "What is the first sound in 'pig'?"
    - Student says: /p/ or /pi/ with short /i/.
    - Scored as: Correct.
- Answered correctly: The correct picture is pointed to that corresponds to the sound given.
  - *Example:* "Which one begins with /b/?"
    - Student points to: picture of ball.
    - Scored as: Correct.
- Self-corrections within 5 seconds: Words mispronounced initially but corrected within 5 seconds and pictures pointed to incorrectly but corrected within 5 seconds.
  - *Example:* "What is the first sound in /skate/?"
    - Student says: /k/ (3 seconds) . . . /sk/.
    - Scored as: Correct.
  - *Example:* "Which one begins with /r/?"
    - Student points to: tree (4 seconds) . . . points to rake.
    - Scored as: Correct
- Dialect/articulation: Variations in pronunciation explainable by local language norms or speech sound production.
  - *Example:* "What is the first sound in 'pen'?"
    - Student says: /pi/ with short /i/.
    - Scored as: Correct.
- Repetitions: Repeating the sound or pointing to the stimuli more than once.
  - *Example:* "What is the first sound in 'sit'?"
    - Student says: /s/ /s/ /s/.
    - Scored as: Correct.
  - *Example:* "Which one begins with /z/?"
    - Student points to: zebra and touches the picture more than once.
    - Scored as: Correct.
- Insertions: Adding the schwa sound.
  - *Example:* "What is the first sound in 'cub'?"
    - Student says: /ku/.
    - Scored as: Correct.

SCORED AS ERRORS

All errors are marked by checking incorrect (0) on the score sheet.

- Mispronunciations/substitutions: When a sound is said incorrectly or is substituted with another sound or when the incorrect stimulus is pointed to.
  - *Example:* "What is the first sound in 'fish'?"
    - Student says: /l/ or /li/ with short /i/.
    - Scored as: Incorrect.

- ■ *Example:* "Which one begins with /s/?"
  - ○ Student points to: picture of train.
  - ○ Scored as: Incorrect.
- • Hesitations without response: Not responding for 5 seconds and being prompted by having the next question read.
  - ■ *Example:* "What's the first sound in 'van'?"
    - ○ Student says: (hesitates for 5 seconds)
    - ○ Scored as: Incorrect and read next question.
- • Hesitations with response: Starting to respond but not finishing by 5 seconds and being prompted by having the next question read.
  - ■ *Example:* "What's the first sound in 'sun'?"
    - ○ Student says: "/k/ no /n/ no /t/." (5 seconds)
    - ○ Scored as: Incorrect and read next question.
  - ■ *Example:* "Which one begins with /m/?"
    - ○ Student points to: every picture on the page until 5 seconds are up.
    - ○ Scored as: Incorrect and read next question.

Special Administration and Scoring Considerations for Onset Sounds CBM

1. Correction procedure: If the student makes an error, he is not corrected.
2. Discontinuation rule: If the student does not get any correct in the first four items, stop and mark all items as incorrect.
3. Elongation of sounds: If the student elongates the sounds and each sound is clearly heard, it is scored as correct.
4. Mismatch between what it said and what is pointed to: If the student says the correct name for a picture but points to the wrong picture, it is scored as correct as long as the starting sounds match the target word.

PHONEME SEGMENTING CBM

Phoneme Segmenting CBM is designed to assess phonemic awareness, specifically the ability to hear a spoken word and produce each individual sound in that word.

Materials Needed to Conduct Phoneme Segmenting CBM

1. Different but equivalent stimuli sheets (teacher/examiner copies).
2. Directions for administering and scoring Phoneme Segmenting CBM.
3. A writing utensil and clipboard or computer to enter student responses.
4. A stopwatch or countdown timer that displays seconds.
5. A quiet testing environment to work with students.
6. An equal-interval graph or a graphing program to plot the data.

Phoneme Segmenting CBM Sheets

Phoneme Segmenting CBM sheets should have a list of words for the teacher/examiner to read, while the student does not have any materials in front of him or her. Each publisher (i.e., aimsweb, DIBELS, EasyCBM, and FastBridge Learning) has a phoneme segmenting task, and they are all given in a similar way. For the purposes of discussing the directions, scoring, and additional considerations, we will be referring to the DIBELS materials. We recommend readers look at the specific measures they will be using to ensure they follow the administration and scoring rules applicable for that specific measure, as there are variations among publishers.

We recommend administering all universal screening assessments in one testing session to save setup time and for consistency in obtaining an accurate score, but it can occur across consecutive days if needed. If three samples of the same CBM task are to be administered, then the median score is used for the final score and can also be placed as the first data point on the student's graph. After that, 20–30 different but equivalent sheets will be used to monitor student progress in reading throughout the year.

Phoneme segmenting must be administered individually. One copy of the sheet will be needed. The student does not have any materials in front of him, and the teacher/examiner should either have a copy of the Phoneme Segmenting CBM sheet in front of her on the computer screen or a paper copy to write on and a writing utensil, as well as a timer and the directions. See Figure 3.3 for an example of the teacher/examiner sheet.

Directions and Scoring Procedures for Phoneme Segmenting CBM

For your convenience, Appendix B includes a reproducible version of the directions and scoring rules for phoneme segmenting.

Directions for Phoneme Segmenting CBM[2]

1. Place the teacher/examiner copy on the clipboard so the student cannot see it.
2. Say: *"We are going to say the sounds in words. Listen to me say all the sounds in the word 'fan': /f/ /a/ /n/. Listen to another word* (pause): *'jump': /j/ /u/ /m/ /p/. Your turn. Say all the sounds in 'soap.'"*
   a. If correct, say: *"Very good saying all the sounds in 'soap.'"* Begin testing.
   b. If incorrect, say: *"I said 'soap,' so you say /s/ /oa/ /p/. Your turn. Say all the sounds in 'soap.'"*
   c. If correct, say: *"Good."* Begin testing.
   d. If incorrect, say: *"OK."* Begin testing.
3. To begin testing, say: *"I am going to say more words. I will say the word and you say all the sounds in the word."*

---

[2] Adapted with permission from DIBELS.

DIBELS® Phoneme Segmentation Fluency

				Score
boat /b/ /oa/ /t/	log /l/ /o/ /g/	stuff /s/ /t/ /u/ /f/	judge /j/ /u/ /j/	10 /13
black /b/ /l/ /a/ /k/	cane /k/ /a/ /n/	verbs /v/ /ir/ /b/ /z/	near /n/ /ea/ /r/	11 /14
run /r/ /u/ /n/	seeds /s/ /ea/ /d/ /z/	have /h/ /a/ /v/	much /m/ /u/ /ch/	10 /13
clue /k/ /l/ /oo/	wet /w/ /e/ /t/	met /m/ /e/ /t/	new /n/ /oo/	9 /11
hill /h/ /i/ /l/	groups /g/ /r/ /oo/ /p/ /s/	knife /n/ /ie/ /f/	bill /b/ /i/ /l/	6 /14
shake /sh/ /ai/ /k/	plane /p/ /l/ /ai/ /n/	own /oa/ /n/	ball /b/ /o/ /l/	/12

Total: __46__

PSF Response Patterns:

☐ Repeats word

☐ Makes random errors

☐ Says initial sound only

☐ Says onset rime

☐ Does not segment blends

☐ Adds sounds

☐ Makes consistent errors on specific sound(s)

☒ Other *some difficulty on vowel sounds and ending sounds*

FIGURE 3.3. Example of teacher/examiner Phoneme Segmenting CBM sheet. Reprinted with permission from DIBELS.

4. Say the first word on the list and then start the timer.
5. Stop the timer after 1 minute and put a bracket after the last sound the student says.

Scoring Phoneme Segmenting CBM

Submit the results using the online system. Or:

1. Count the total number of items attempted.
2. Count the total number of errors.
3. Calculate rate: Total items attempted – total errors = total correct per minute.
4. Calculate accuracy: Total correct ÷ total items attempted = percent correct.

SCORED AS CORRECT

Phoneme Segmenting CBM is scored based on each different, correct, part of the word that is said. Each correct part is underlined and counted as a correct sound segment.

- Pronounced correctly: Each sound segment is pronounced correctly.
  - *Example: trip*
    - Student says: /t/ /r/ /i/ /p/.
    - Scored as: <u>t</u> <u>r</u> <u>i</u> <u>p</u> = 4 correct sounds.
    - Student says: /tr/ /i/ /p/.
    - Scored as: <u>t r</u> <u>i</u> <u>p</u> = 3 correct sounds.
    - Student says: /tr/ /ip/.
    - Scored as: <u>t r</u> <u>i p</u> = 2 correct sounds.
    - Student says: /tr/ /rip/.
    - Scored as: <u>t r i p</u> = 2 correct sounds.
- Self-corrections within 3 seconds: Segments mispronounced initially but corrected within 3 seconds.
  - *Example: dug*
    - Student says: /d/ /i/ (2 seconds) /u/ /g/.
    - Scored as: <u>d</u> u̶ <u>g</u> = 3 correct sounds.
- Dialect/articulation: Variations in pronunciation explainable by local language norms or speech sound production.
  - *Example: late*
    - Student says: /w/ /ai/ /t/.
    - Scored as: <u>l</u> <u>a</u> <u>te</u> = 3 correct sounds.
- Repetitions: Repeating the same sound more than once.
  - *Example: sat*
    - Student says: /s/ /s/ /s/ /a/ /a/ /t/.
    - Scored as: <u>s</u> <u>a</u> <u>t</u> = 3 correct sounds.
- Insertions: Adding sounds to the beginning, middle, or end of the word or the schwa sound.
  - *Example: pot*
    - Student says: /s/ /p/ /o/ /t/.

    or
    - Student says: /p/ /f/ /o/ /t/.

    or
    - Student says: /p/ /o/ /t/ /s/.
    - Scored as: <u>p</u> <u>o</u> <u>t</u> = 3 correct sounds.
  - *Example: kick*
    - Student says: /ku/ /i/ /ku/.
    - Scored as: <u>k</u> <u>i</u> <u>ck</u> = 3 correct sounds.

SCORED AS ERRORS

All errors are marked by drawing a line through the mispronounced sound(s). Sounds that are not produced are left blank. If the student does not segment the word, the word is circled.

- Mispronunciations/substitutions: When a sound is said incorrectly or substituted with another sound.
  - *Example: bed*
    - ○ Student says: /r/ /e/ /d/ with short /e/.
    - ○ Scored as: ~~b~~ e d = 2 correct sounds.
- Omissions: Sounds that are not produced.
  - *Example: boat*
    - ○ Student says: /oa/ /t/.
    - ○ Scored as: b oa t = 2 correct sounds.
- Hesitations without response: Not responding for 3 seconds and being prompted by having the next word read.
  - *Example: moon*
    - ○ Student says: (silent for 3 seconds).
    - ○ Scored as: ~~m oo n~~ = 0 correct sounds and next word is given.
- Hesitations with response: Starting to respond but not finishing by 3 seconds and being prompted by having the next word read.
  - *Example: star*
    - ○ Student says: /st/ (3 seconds).
    - ○ Scored as: s t a r = 1 correct sound and next word is given.
- Reversals: Transposing two or more sounds.
  - *Example: bed*
    - ○ Student says: /d/ /e/ /b/.
    - ○ Scored as: ~~b~~ e ~~d~~ = 1 correct sound.
- Read as whole word: Not segmenting the word into different parts.
  - *Example: trip*
    - ○ Student says: /trip/.
    - ○ Scored as: (t r i p) = 0 correct sounds.

Special Administration and Scoring Considerations for Phoneme Segmenting CBM

1. Correction procedure: If the student makes an error, he is not corrected.
2. Discontinuation rule: If the student does not get any correct sounds in the first row, stop and record a score of 0.
3. Finish before 1 minute: If the student finishes in less than 1 minute, note the number of seconds it took to complete the sheet/list and prorate the score. The formula for prorating is:

$$\frac{\text{Total number of correct sounds}}{\text{Number of seconds it took to finish}} \times 60 = \text{Estimated number of correct sounds}$$

Example: The student finished the CBM sheet in just 50 seconds and got 20 sounds correct.

$$\frac{20}{50} \times 60 = 0.4 \times 60 = 24$$

We estimate that the student would have produced approximately 24 sounds correctly in 1 minute had we provided more words and timed the student for the full 1 minute.

4. If the student elongates the sounds and each sound is clearly heard, it is scored as correct.

LETTER NAMING CBM

Letter Naming CBM does not assess phonological awareness or decoding; rather, it is used as a risk indicator for reading because it measures automaticity. This task is similar to other rapid naming tasks that do not use letters but instead ask the student to quickly name colors, numbers, or objects. This task is included here because it is a common CBM assessment often included in a composite score for universal screening. While we want students to be able to name the letters, the skill that is more closely related to decoding and reading is knowing the *sounds* of the letters. Given the choice, we would encourage teachers to use Letter Naming CBM only when it is included with other reading measures for universal screening. For the purposes of progress monitoring, we would support only the use of Letter Sounds CBM, which is also described in detail below.

Materials Needed to Conduct Letter Naming CBM

1. Different but equivalent stimuli sheets (student and teacher/examiner copies).
2. Directions for administering and scoring Letter Naming CBM.
3. A writing utensil and clipboard or computer to enter student responses.
4. A stopwatch or countdown timer that displays seconds.
5. A quiet testing environment to work with students.
6. An equal-interval graph or a graphing program to plot the data.

Letter Naming CBM Sheets

Letter Naming CBM sheets should have different items (or sequences of items) and should have at least 26 letters per sheet. The best way to accomplish this is to purchase or obtain generic sheets that have been developed specially for collecting letter names. For the purposes of discussing the directions, scoring, and additional considerations, we will be referring to the DIBELS materials. We recommend that readers look at the specific measures they will be using to ensure they follow the administration and scoring rules applicable for that specific measure, as there are variations among publishers.

We recommend administering all universal screening assessments in one testing session to save setup time and for consistency in obtaining an accurate score, but it can occur across consecutive days if needed. If three samples of the same CBM task are to be administered, then the median score is used for the final score and can also be placed as the first data point on the student's graph. We would not recommend obtaining additional but equivalent sheets for the purpose of monitoring student progress but would instead encourage readers to use Letter Sounds CBM or another task aligned with the students' skills and the instruction they are receiving.

Letter Naming CBM must be administered individually. Two copies of the sheet will be needed. The student should have a copy of the letter names in front of her, and the teacher/examiner should either have a copy of the letter names sheet in front of him on the computer screen or a paper copy to write on and a writing utensil, as well as a timer and the directions. See Figures 3.4 and 3.5 for examples of each type of sheet.

Directions and Scoring Procedures for Letter Naming CBM

For your convenience, Appendix B includes a reproducible version of the directions and scoring rules for Letter Naming CBM.

Directions for Letter Naming CBM[3]

1. Place the copy of the student sheet in front of the student.
2. Place the teacher/examiner copy on the clipboard so the student cannot see it.
3. Say: *"I am going to show you some letters. I want you to point to each letter and say its name."* (Put the page of letters in front of the student.)
4. To begin testing say: *"Start here (point to the first letter at the top of the page). Go this way (sweep your finger across the first two rows of letters) and say each letter name. Put your finger under the first letter (point). Ready, begin."*
5. Start the timer after you say: *"Begin."*
6. Stop the timer after 1 minute and bracket the last letter named.

Scoring Letter Naming CBM

Submit the results using the online system. Or:

1. Count the total number of items attempted.
2. Count the total number of errors.
3. Calculate rate: Total items attempted – total errors = total correct per minute.
4. Calculate accuracy: Total correct ÷ total items attempted = percent correct.

---

[3] Adapted with permission from DIBELS.

▶ s	J	z	v	e	X	T	t	V	D
f	F	W	Q	P	q	l	c	O	o
R	n	B	w	g	E	d	u	p	y
S	m	x	L	k	Z	a	Y	H	j
i	K	U	M	G	r	A	N	h	C
I	b	S	F	f	u	L	A	m	B
V	T	Y	G	e	W	E	a	N	X
l	b	M	C	q	z	P	x	i	Q
g	J	O	s	d	Z	K	o	v	j
D	t	h	w	R	U	c	r	I	k
n	H	y	p	s	J	z	v	e	X

FIGURE 3.4. Example of student Letter Naming CBM sheet. Reprinted with permission from DIBELS.

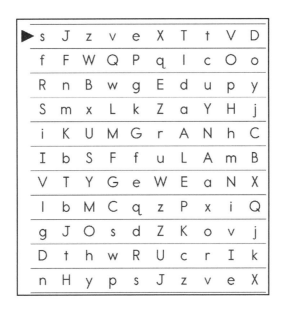

1 DIBELS® Letter Naming Fluency
Grade K/Benchmark 1

▶ s	J	z	v	e	X	T	t	V	D
f	F	W	Q	P	q	l	c	O	o
R	n	B	w	g	E	d	u	p	y
S	m	x	L	k	Z	a	Y	H	j
i	K	U	M	G	r	A	N	h	C
I	b	S	F	f	u	L	A	m	B
V	T	Y	G	e	W	E	a	N	X
l	b	M	C	q	z	P	x	i	Q
g	J	O	s	d	Z	K	o	v	j
D	t	h	w	R	U	c	r	I	k
n	H	y	p	s	J	z	v	e	X

Total Correct: _____

LNF Response Patterns:

☐ Makes random errors   ☐ Doesn't track correctly
☐ Makes consistent errors on specific letter(s) ☐ Other
☐ Says letter sound instead of letter name

FIGURE 3.5. Example of teacher/examiner Letter Naming CBM sheet. Reprinted with permission from DIBELS.

SCORED AS CORRECT

Letter Naming CBM is scored based on each correct pronunciation of the individual names of the letters. Each correct letter is counted toward total correct letter names; only errors and self-corrections are marked on the sheet.

- Pronounced correctly: Each letter must be named correctly.
    - *Example: E, h, t, S, f, r, q, H, I, v*
        - Student says: *E, H, T, S, F, R, Q, H, I, V.*
        - Scored as: *E, h, t, S, f, r, q, H, I, v* = 10 correct letter names.
- Self-corrections within 3 seconds: Letter names mispronounced initially but corrected within 3 seconds.
    - *Example: E, h, t, S, f, r, q, H, I, v*
        - Student says: *E, K* (2 seconds), *H, T, S, F, R, Q, H, I, V.*
        - Scored as: *E, $\cancel{h}$, t, S, f, r, q, H, I, v* = 10 correct letter names.
- Dialect/articulation: Variations in pronunciation explainable by local language norms or speech sound production.
    - *Example: E, h, t, S, f, r, q, H, I, v*
        - Student says: *E, H, T, S, THeef, Waar, Q, H, I, V.*
        - Scored as: *E, h, t, S, f, r, q, H, I, v* = 10 correct letter names.
- Repetitions: Repeating the letter name more than once.
    - *Example: E, h, t, S, f, r, q, H, I, v*
        - Student says: *E, E, H, H, T, T, S, F, R, Q, H, I, V.*
        - Scored as: *E, h, t, S, f, r, q, H, I, v* = 10 correct letter names.

SCORED AS ERRORS

All errors are marked by drawing a line through the mispronounced or skipped letter.

- Mispronunciations/substitutions: When a letter is named incorrectly.
    - *Example: E, h, t, S, f, r, q, H, I, v*
        - Student says: *E, K, T, YES, F, R, Q, H, I, W.*
        - Scored as: *E, $\cancel{h}$, t, $\cancel{S}$, f, r, q, H, I, $\cancel{v}$* = 7 correct letter names.
- Omissions: Letters that are not produced.
    - *Example: E, h, t, S, f, r, q, H, I, v*
        - Student says: *E, H, T, S, R, Q, H, V.*
        - Scored as: *E, h, t, S, $\cancel{f}$, r, q, H, $\cancel{I}$, v* = 8 correct letter names.
- Hesitations without response: Not responding for 3 seconds and being prompted by providing the name of that letter.
    - *Example: E, h, t, S, f, r, q, H, I, v*
        - Student says: *E, H, T,* (3 seconds. *You say S), F, R,* (3 seconds. *You say Q), H, I, V.*
        - Scored as: *E, h, t, $\cancel{S}$, f, r, $\cancel{q}$, H, I, v* = 8 correct letter names.

- Hesitations with response: Starting to respond but not finishing by 3 seconds and being prompted by providing the name of that letter.
  - *Example: E, h, t, S, f, r, q, H, I, v*
    - Student says: *E, H, T, (eeSSS, 3 seconds) (You say S), F, R, Q, H, I, V.*
    - Scored as: *E, h, t, S̶, f, r, q, H, I, v* = 9 correct letter names.
- Reversals: Transposing two or more letters.
  - *Example: E, h, t, S, f, r, q, H, I, v*
    - Student says: *E, H, T, S, R, F, Q, H, I, V.*
    - Scored as: *E, h, t, S, f̶, r̶, q, H, I, v* = 8 correct letter names.

Special Administration and Scoring Considerations for Letter Naming CBM

1. Correction procedure: If the student makes an error, he is not corrected. The only time a letter name is provided is if the student hesitates for 3 seconds.
2. Skip a row: If the student skips a row, draw a line through it and do *not* count that row in scoring.
3. Discontinuation rule: If the student does not get any correct within the first row (10 letters), discontinue the task and record a score of 0.
4. Finish before 1 minute: If the student finishes in less than 1 minute, she receives the score obtained. Scores are *not* prorated for this measure.
5. Confusion of similar-looking letters: If the student says "I" or "L" for the uppercase "I," both are scored correct.
6. Says letter sound for letter name: If the student says letter sounds, say: **"Say the letter name, not its sound."** (Use only once.)
7. Does not answer from left to right: If the student moves from right to left say: **"Go this way."** Sweep your finger across the row. (Use only once.)
8. Loses his place: If a student loses his place on the page, point to the items he is on. (Use as often as needed.)

LETTER SOUNDS CBM

Letter Sounds CBM is designed to assess the most common sounds associated with the 26 letters of the alphabet, with the short sound represented for the vowels.

Materials Needed to Conduct Letter Sounds CBM

1. Different but equivalent reading sheets (student and teacher/examiner copies).
2. Directions for administering and scoring Letter Sound CBM.
3. A writing utensil and clipboard or computer to enter student responses.
4. A stopwatch or countdown timer that displays seconds.

5. A quiet testing environment to work with students.
6. An equal-interval graph or a graphing program to plot the data.

Letter Sounds CBM Reading Sheets

Letter Sounds CBM reading sheets should have different items (or sequences of items) and should have at least 26 letters per sheet. The best way to accomplish this is to purchase or obtain generic sheets that have been developed specifically for collecting Letter Sounds CBM data. For the purposes of discussing the directions, scoring, and additional considerations we will be referring to aimsweb. We recommend people look at specific measures they will be using to ensure they follow the administration and scoring rules applicable for that specific measure, as there are variations among publishers.

We recommend administering all universal screening assessments in one testing session to save setup time and for consistency in obtaining an accurate score, but it can occur across consecutive days if needed. If three samples of the same CBM task are to be administered, then the median score is used for the final score and can also be placed as the first data point on the student's graph. After that, 20–30 different but equivalent sheets will be used to monitor student progress in reading throughout the year.

Letter Sounds CBM must be administered individually. Two copies of the sheet will be needed. The student should have a copy of the Letter Sounds CBM sheet in front of him, and the teacher/examiner should either have a copy of the Letter Sounds CBM sheet in front of her on the computer screen or a paper copy to write on and a writing utensil, as well as a timer and the directions. See Figures 3.6 and 3.7 for examples of each type of sheet.

Directions and Scoring Procedures for Letter Sounds CBM

For your convenience, Appendix B includes a reproducible version of the directions and scoring rules for Letter Sounds CBM.

Directions for Letter Sounds CBM[4]

1. Place the copy of the student sheet in front of the student.
2. Place the teacher/examiner copy on the clipboard so the student cannot see it.
3. Say: *"**Here are some letters** (point to the student copy). **Begin here** (point to the first letter) **and tell me the sounds of as many letters as you can. If you come to a letter you don't know, I'll tell it to you. Are there any questions? Put your finger under the first letter. Ready? Begin."** (Trigger stopwatch or timer for 1 minute.)*
4. Follow along on the teacher/examiner copy as the student reads and puts a slash (/) through any incorrect letters.
5. At the end of 1 minute say: *"**Thank you**"* and put a bracket (]) after the last sound provided.

---

[4]Adapted with permission from aimsweb (Shinn & Shinn, 2002a).

t	d	n	r	p	c	z	v	w	k
m	b	t	f	v	z	i	c	d	p
v	y	e	l	b	j	s	t	f	a
c	n	f	r	m	b	t	h	z	s
j	k	p	s	f	h	i	r	o	m
s	z	p	i	j	r	e	d	g	o
j	g	a	t	s	h	c	r	k	l
j	u	k	y	a	s	z	e	i	v
m	s	d	g	f	l	b	v	j	c
t	e	m	l	w	j	y	z	f	v

FIGURE 3.6. Example of student Letter Sounds CBM sheet. From aimsweb (2003). Reprinted with permission from Edformation, Inc.

Given To: _____   Given By: _____   Date: _____

t d n r p c z v w k   /10 (10)

m b t f v z i c d p   /10 (20)

v y e l b j s t f a   /10 (30)

c n f r m b t h z s   /10 (40)

j k p s f h i r o m   /10 (50)

s z p i j r e d g o   /10 (60)

j g a t s h c r k l   /10 (70)

j u k y a s z e i v   /10 (80)

m s d g f l b v j c   /10 (90)

t e m l w j y z f v   /10 (100)

                                                          /

FIGURE 3.7. Example of teacher/examiner Letter Sounds CBM sheet. From aimsweb (2003). Reprinted with permission from Edformation, Inc.

Scoring Letter Sounds CBM

Submit the results using the online system. Or:

1. Count the total number of items attempted.
2. Count the total number of errors.
3. Calculate rate: Total items attempted – total errors = total correct per minute.
4. Calculate accuracy: Total correct ÷ total items attempted = percent correct.

SCORED AS CORRECT

Letter Sounds CBM is scored based on pronouncing the most common sound of the letter correctly. Each correct sound is counted toward total correct letter sounds; only errors are marked on the sheet. A pronunciation key for the most common sounds is provided in Table 3.2.

- Pronounced correctly: The sound must be pronounced correctly. Short vowel (not long vowel) sounds are considered correct.
  - *Example*: a, e, i, o, u
    - Student says: /a/ (like *apple*), /e/ (like *echo*), /i/ (like *itch*), /o/ (like *octopus*), /u/ (like *up*).
    - Scored as: *a, e, i, o, u* = 5 correct letter sounds.
- Self-corrections within 3 seconds: Sounds mispronounced initially but corrected within 3 seconds are scored as correct and *sc* is written above the letter.
  - *Example*: a
    - Student says: long /a/ sound as in *ape* (2 seconds) . . . short /a/ sound as in *apple*.
    - Scored as: *a* = 1 correct letter sound.

TABLE 3.2. Most Common Sounds Pronunciation Key

Letter	Example	Letter	Example
a	apple	l	lip
e	echo	m	mat
i	itch	n	not
o	octopus	p	pat
u	up	q	quick
b	big	r	rat
c	cat	s	sit
d	dad	t	top
f	fat	v	van
g	go	w	will
h	hat	x	ox
j	jump	y	yell
k	kit	z	zip

- Dialect/articulation: Variations in pronunciation explainable by local language norms or speech sound production.
  - *Example*: s
    - Student says: /th/ instead of /s/. This would be accepted if due to an articulation problem.
    - Scored as: *s* = 1 correct letter sound.
- Repetitions: Repeating the sound more than once.
  - *Example: s, d, w*
    - Student says: /s/ /s/ /d/ /w/.
    - Scored as: *s, d, w* = 3 correct letter sounds.
- Insertions: Adding the schwa sound.
  - *Example: b, t, m*
    - Student says: /buh/ /tuh/ /muh/.
    - Scored as: *b, t, m* = 3 correct letter sounds.

SCORED AS ERRORS

All errors are marked by drawing a line through the misprounced or skipped letter.

- Mispronunciations/substitutions: When a letter sound is either mispronounced or substituted with other letter sounds.
  - *Example*: p
    - Student says: /b/.
    - Scored as: p̸ = 0 correct letter sound.
- Omissions: Letter sounds that are not produced.
  - *Example: t, d, n, r, p, c, i, l*
    - Student says: /t/ /d/ /n/ /p/ /c/ /i/ /l/.
    - Scored as: *t, d, n, r̸, p, c, i, l* = 7 correct letter sounds.
- Hesitations without response: Not responding for 3 seconds and being prompted by providing the sound of that letter.
  - *Example: t, d, n, r, p, c, i, l*
    - Student says: /t/ /d/ /n/ /r/ /p/ /c/ (hesitates 3 seconds on *i*). Say: "/i/." Point to next letter and say: **"What sound?"** /l/.
    - Scored as: *t, d, n, r, p, c, i̸, l* = 7 correct letter sounds.
- Reversals: Transposing two or more sounds.
  - *Example: t, d, n, r, c, p, i, l*
    - Student says: /t/ /d/ /n/ /c/ /r/ /p/ /i/ /l/.
    - Scored as: *t, d, n, r̸, c̸, p, i, l* = 6 correct letter sounds.

*Special Administration and Scoring Considerations
for Letter Sounds CBM*

1. Correction procedure: If the student makes an error, he is not corrected. The only time a letter sound is provided is if the student hesitates for 3 seconds.
2. Skip an entire row: If the student skips a row, draw a line through it and do *not* count it in the scoring as attempted or as errors.
3. Discontinuation rule: If the student does not get any sounds correct in the first row, discontinue the task.

   If the student says the letter *name* instead of the letter *sound*, say: ***"Remember to tell me the sound the letter makes, not its name."*** This is provided *one time* only.
4. If the student finishes in less than 1 minute, note the number of seconds it took to complete the sheet/list and prorate the score. The formula for prorating is:

$$\frac{\text{Total number of correct sounds}}{\text{Number of seconds it took to finish}} \times 60 = \text{Estimated number of correct sounds}$$

   Example: The student finished the sheet in just 48 seconds and got 24 sounds correct.

$$\frac{24}{48} \times 60 = 0.5 \times 60 = 30$$

   We estimate that the student would have read approximately 30 letter sounds correctly in 1 minute had we provided more letters and timed the student for the full 1 minute.
5. Elongation of sounds: If the student elongates the sounds and each sound is clearly heard, it is scored as correct.
6. The capital letter *I* and lowercase *L* look alike, so either sound is considered correct.

NONSENSE WORDS CBM

Nonsense Words CBM is a direct measure of basic decoding skills. The task uses nonsense words in order to eliminate the chance the student may have memorized or learned the words already. The only way the student can successfully read these words is by applying their knowledge of letter–sound correspondences and the ability to blend the sounds together into words. While you would *not* want to teach children nonsense words, since every real word they encounter that is unknown to them is nonsense, this task provides reliable information related to reading words by applying what one knows about letter–sound relations.

Materials Needed to Conduct Nonsense Words CBM

1. Different but equivalent reading sheets (student and teacher/examiner copies).
2. Directions for administering and scoring Nonsense Words CBM.

3. A writing utensil and clipboard or computer to enter student responses.
4. A stopwatch or countdown timer that displays seconds.
5. A quiet testing environment to work with students.
6. An equal-interval graph or a graphing program to plot the data.

Nonsense Words CBM Sheets

Nonsense Words CBM sheets should have different items (or sequences of items) and should consist of at least 50 words each. The best way to accomplish this is to purchase or obtain generic sheets that have been developed specifically for collecting Nonsense Words CBM data. For the purposes of discussing the directions, scoring, and additional considerations we will be referring to the FastBridge Learning materials. We recommend readers look at the specific measures they will be using to ensure they follow the administration and scoring rules applicable for that specific measure, as there are variations among publishers.

We recommend administering all universal screening assessments in one testing session to save setup time and for consistency in obtaining an accurate score, but it can occur across consecutive days if needed. If three samples of the same CBM task are to be administered, then the median score is used for the final score and can also be placed as the first data point on the student's graph. After that, 20–30 different but equivalent sheets will be used to monitor student progress in reading throughout the year.

Nonsense Words CBM must be administered individually. Two copies of the sheet will be needed. The student should have a copy of the Nonsense Words CBM sheet in front of him, and the teacher/examiner should either have a copy of the Nonsense Words CBM sheet in front of him on the computer screen or a paper copy to write on and a writing utensil, as well as a timer and the directions. See Figures 3.8 and 3.9 for examples of each type of sheet.

Directions and Scoring Procedures for Nonsense Words CBM

For your convenience, Appendix B includes a reproducible version of the directions and scoring rules for Nonsense Words CBM.

Directions for Nonsense Words CBM[5]

1. Place the copy of the practice page in front of the student.
2. Place the teacher/examiner copy on the clipboard or pull up the scoring sheet on the computer screen so the student cannot see it.
3. Say: *"I am going to have you read some pretend words. An example of a pretend word is 'tup'* (point to the word "tup"). *If you cannot say the word, you can say the sounds in the word: /t/ /u/ /p/* (point to each letter in the word). *When you read these words, try to say the whole word. If you don't know how to say it, then you can say the sounds of each letter instead."*

---

[5]Adapted with permission from FastBridge Learning.

FIGURE 3.8. Example of student Nonsense Words CBM sheet. Reprinted with permission from FastBridge Learning.

FIGURE 3.9. Example of teacher/examiner Nonsense Words CBM sheet. Reprinted with permission from FastBridge Learning.

4. Say: *"Now you try. Read this pretend word"* (*point to "pof"*).
   a. If the student reads as whole word, say: *"Good! The letters 'P', 'O', and 'F' make the pretend word 'POF.'"* Begin directions for test.
   b. If the student reads the sounds, say: *"Good! The letter sounds in 'POF' are /p/ /o/ /f/."* Begin directions for test.
   c. If incorrect, say: *"The pretend word is 'POF': /p/ /o/ /f/—'POF.' When you say the sounds together the pretend word is 'POF.' The sounds in 'POF' are /p/ /o/ /f/. Remember you can say the individual letter sounds OR the whole word."* Begin directions for test.
5. To begin the test say: *"Now here is a list of more pretend words for you to read. When I say 'Begin' start reading the pretend words out loud here* (*point to the first word*). *Read across the page, then go to the next line* (*point to demonstrate*). *Try to say each one as a whole word. If you can't say it as a whole word, then try to sound out the letters."*
6. Say: *"OK? So what are you going to do?"* (*Have the student tell you how she can say the whole nonsense word OR the sounds in the words—not both. Clarify if needed*). *"Good."*
7. Say: *"Ready? Begin."* (*Start timer when student says the first nonsense word.*)
8. Follow along on the teacher/examiner copy and click on words that are said incorrectly if using the computer version, or for the paper/pencil version put a slash (/) through any incorrect nonsense words. (The test is not scored at the sound level, so if the student is reading it sound for sound the entire word is still the unit for scoring purposes.)
9. At the end of 1 minute say *"Stop"* and put a bracket (]) after the last word read.

Scoring Nonsense Words CBM

Submit the results using the online system. Or:

1. Count the total number of items attempted.
2. Count the total number of errors.
3. Calculate rate: Total items attempted – total errors = total correct per minute.
4. Calculate accuracy: Total correct ÷ total items attempted = percent correct.

SCORED AS CORRECT

Nonsense Words CBM is scored based on pronouncing the most common sound of the letter correctly either letter-by-letter or blended together and read as an entire word. Vowel sounds: Short vowel (not long vowel) sounds are considered correct along with the most common sound for the consonants. You can refer back to Table 3.2, the Most Common Sounds Pronunciation Key, for assistance with the correct sounds.

- Pronounced correctly: The sounds must be pronounced correctly in isolation or blended into words.
  - *Example*: *kiv, hoz, ruc, af, bix*
    - Student says: /k/ /i/ /v/, /ho/ /z/, /ruc/, /af/, /b/ /ix/.
    - Scored as: *kiv, hoz, ruc, af, bix* = 5 correct nonsense words.

- Self-corrections: Sounds or words mispronounced initially but corrected within 3 seconds are scored as correct and *sc* is written above the word or if using the computer screen the word is clicked on again to remove the highlighting.
  - *Example*: *nus, yif, jex, ut, tok, zam*
    - Student says: /nut/ (2 seconds, /nus/), /yif/, /jex/, /ut/, /took/ (2 seconds, /tok/), /zam/.
    - Scored as: *nus, yif, jex, ut, tok, zam* = 6 correct nonsense words.
- Dialect/articulation: Variations in pronunciation explainable by local language norms or speech sound production.
  - *Example*: *nus*
    - Student says: /nuth/ and gives the /th/ instead of /s/ due to an articulation issue.
    - Scored as: *nus* = 1 correct nonsense word.
- Repetitions: Repeating the word more than once.
  - *Example*: *kov, yef, rup*
    - Student says: /k/ /k/ /ov/, /yef/, /yef/, /rup/.
    - Scored as: *kov, yef, rup* = 3 correct nonsense words.

SCORED AS ERRORS

All errors are marked by drawing a slash through the word or clicking on the word so that it is highlighted with the computer version.

- Mispronunciations/substitutions: Letter sounds or words either mispronounced or substituted with other letter sounds.
  - *Example*: *nus, yif, jex, ut, tok, zam*
    - Student says: /nus/, /yip/, /jex/, /at/, /tok/, /sam/.
    - Scored as: *nus, yif, jex, ut, tok, zam* = 3 correct nonsense words.
- Omissions: Letter sounds or words that are not produced.
  - *Example*: *nus, yif, jex, ut, tok, zam*
    - Student says: /ns/, /yip/, /jex/, /at/, /tk/, /zm/.
    - Scored as: *nus, yif, jex, ut, tok, zam* = 2 correct nonsense words.
- Hesitations without response: Not responding for 3 seconds and being prompted by providing the sound or word.
  - *Example*: *nus, yif, jex, ut, tok, zam*
    - Student says: /n/ (3 seconds; say /u/), /yif/, /jex/, /ut/, (3 seconds; say "tok"), /zam/.
    - Scored as: *nus, yif, jex, ut, tok, zam* = 4 correct nonsense words.
- Hesitations with response: Starting to respond but not finishing by 3 seconds and being prompted by providing the sound or word.
  - *Example*: *nus, yif, jex, ut, tok, zam*
    - Student says: /nnnnnnnn/ (3 seconds; say /u/), /yif/, /jex/, /uuuuuuuuu/ (3 seconds; say "ut"), /tok/, /zam./
    - Scored as: *nus, yif, jex, ut, tok, zam* = 4 correct nonsense words.
- Reversals: Transposing two or more sounds or words.
  - *Example*: *nus, yif, jex, ut, tok, zam*
    - Student says: /n/ /u/ /s/, /y/ /f/ /i/, /jex/, /tok/, /ut/, /zam/.
    - Scored as: *nus, yif, jex, ut, tok, zam* = 3 correct nonsense words.

Special Administration and Scoring Considerations for Nonsense Words CBM

1. Correction procedure: If the student makes an error, she is not corrected. The only time a letter sound or words is provided is if the student hesitates for 3 seconds.
2. Skip an entire row: If a student skips as entire row, draw a line through it or use the "bulk errors" on the computer scoring and each word in that row is scored as an error.
3. Discontinuation rule: If the student does not get any words correct in the first two rows (10 words), discontinue the task and mark a score of 0.
4. Finish before 1 minute: If the student finishes in less than 1 minute, note the number of seconds it took to complete the sheet/list and prorate the score. If using the computer version it will automatically prorate the score for you. The formula for prorating is:

$$\frac{\text{Total number of correct sounds or words}}{\text{Number of seconds it took to finish}} \times 60 = \text{Estimated number of correct sounds or words}$$

Example: The student finished the sheet in just 55 seconds and got 30 words correct.

$$\frac{30}{55} \times 60 = 0.54 \times 60 = 32$$

We estimate that the student would have read approximately 32 words correctly in 1 minute had we provided more words and timed the student for the full 1 minute.

5. Elongation of sounds: If the student elongates the sounds in the words and each sound is clearly heard, it is scored as correct.
6. Level of scoring: The student is only scored at the word level regardless if he reads the individual sounds in the word or the entire word.

WORD IDENTIFICATION CBM

Word Identification CBM is used to measure student's reading skills related to commonly used words in the early grades. The word list provides an indication of word reading without having to read connected text or sentences.

Materials Needed to Conduct Word Identification CBM

1. Different but equivalent reading sheets (student and teacher/examiner copies).
2. Directions for administering and scoring Word Identification CBM.
3. A writing utensil and clipboard or computer to enter student responses.
4. A stopwatch or countdown timer that displays seconds.
5. A quiet testing environment to work with students.
6. An equal-interval graph or a graphing program to plot the data.

Word Identification CBM Sheets

Word Identification CBM sheets should have different items (or sequences of items) and should consist of at least 50 words each. The reading skills should sample those the student is expected to master throughout the entire school year. The best way to accomplish this is to purchase generic sheets that have been developed specifically for this purpose. For the purposes of discussing the directions, scoring, and additional considerations we will be referring to the Fuchs and Fuchs materials. We recommend readers look at the specific measures they will be using to ensure they follow the administration and scoring rules applicable for that specific measure, as there are variations among publishers.

We recommend administering all universal screening assessments in one testing session to save setup time and for consistency in obtaining an accurate score, but it can occur across consecutive days if needed. If three samples of the same CBM task are to be administered, then the median score is used for the final score and can also be placed as the first data point on the student's graph. After that, 20–30 different but equivalent sheets will be used to monitor student progress in reading throughout the year.

Word Identification CBM must be administered individually. Two copies of the sheet will be needed. The student should have a copy of the Word Identification CBM sheet in front of him, and the teacher/examiner should either have a copy of the Word Identification CBM sheet in front of her on the computer screen or a paper copy to write on and a writing utensil, as well as a timer and the directions. See Figures 3.10 and 3.11 for examples of each type of sheet.

Directions and Scoring Procedure for Word Identification CBM

For your convenience, Appendix B includes a reproducible version of the directions and scoring rules for Word Identification CBM.

Directions for Word Identification CBM[6]

1. Place the copy of the student list in front of the student.
2. Place the teacher/examiner copy on the clipboard so the student cannot see it.
3. Say: ***"When I say 'Begin,' I want you to read these words as quickly and correctly as you can. Start here*** (*point to the first word*) ***and go down the page*** (*run your finger down the first column*). ***If you don't know a word, skip it and try the next word. Keep reading until I say 'Stop.' Do you have any questions? Begin."*** (*Trigger stopwatch or timer for 1 minute.*)
4. Follow along on the teacher/examiner copy as the student reads and *put a slash (/) through any incorrect words.*
5. At the end of 1 minute, say: ***"Stop"*** and put a bracket ( ]) after the last word read.

---

[6]Adapted with permission from Fuchs and Fuchs (2004).

Student:		Date:	
Class:		Correct Items:	
		Total Items Attempted:	

tell	first	write	before
don't	these	work	call
your	because	both	wash
sit	does	very	been
best	their	found	cold
its	those	goes	sing
green	many	right	or
wish	off	sleep	which

FIGURE 3.10. Example of student Word Identification CBM sheet. Reprinted with permission from Intervention Central.

Curriculum-Based Assessment List: Examiner Copy

This answer key contains 32 items from the following assessment list(s):

- *Dolch Words: Second Grade*

Student: _____ Date: _____
Class: _____ Correct Items: _____
Total Items Attempted: _____

Item 1 tell	Item 2 first	Item 3 write	Item 4 before	4/4
Item 5 don't	Item 6 these	Item 7 work	Item 8 call	4/8
Item 9 your	Item 10 because	Item 11 both	Item 12 wash	4/12
Item 13 sit	Item 14 does	Item 15 very	Item 16 been	4/16
Item 17 best	Item 18 their	Item 19 found	Item 20 cold	4/20
Item 21 its	Item 22 those	Item 23 goes	Item 24 sing	4/24
Item 25 green	Item 26 many	Item 27 right	Item 28 or	4/28
Item 20 wish	Item 30 off	Item 31 sleep	Item 32 which	4/32

FIGURE 3.11. Example of teacher/examiner Word Identification CBM sheet. Reprinted with permission from Intervention Central.

Scoring Word Identification CBM

Submit the results using the online system. Or:

1. Count the total number of words attempted in 1 minute.
2. Count the total number of errors.
3. Calculate rate: Total items attempted – total errors = total correct per minute.
4. Calculate accuracy: Total correct ÷ total items attempted = percent correct.

SCORED AS CORRECT

Word Identification CBM is scored based on the correct pronunciation of the entire word.

- Pronounced correctly: The word must be pronounced correctly.
  - *Example*: *made*
    - Student says: /made/.
    - Scored as: *made* = 1 word identified correctly.
- Self-corrections within 3 seconds: Words mispronounced initially but corrected within 3 seconds.
  - *Example*: *where*
    - Student says: /were/ (2 seconds) . . . /where/.
    - Scored as: *where* = 1 word identified correctly.
- Dialect/articulation: Variations in pronunciation explainable by local language norms or speech sound production.
  - *Example*: *either*
    - Student says: /either/ with a long /i/ or long /e/.
    - Scored as: *either* = 1 word identified correctly.
- Repetitions: Repeating the word more than once.
  - *Example*: *what, have, name*
    - Student says: /what/ /what/ /have/ /name/.
    - Scored as: *what, have, name* = 3 words identified correctly.

SCORED AS ERRORS

All errors are marked with a slash (╱)through the word.

- Mispronunciations/substitutions: Words either mispronounced or substituted with other words.
  - *Example*: *mother*
    - Student says: /mom/.
    - Scored as: *mother* = 0 word identified correctly.

- Omissions: Words that are not produced.
    - *Example*: *and, as, at, one, said, into, could*
        - Student says: /and/ /as/ /one/ /said/ /into/ /could/.
        - Scored as: *and, as, ~~at~~, one, said, into, could* = 6 words identified correctly.
- Hesitations without response: Not responding for 2 seconds and being prompted by pointing to the next word and saying "**What word?**"
    - *Example*: *and, as, at, one, said, into, could*
        - Student says: /and/ /as/ /at/ (hesitates 2 seconds on *one*). Point to *said* and say: "**What word?**" /said/ /into/ /could/.
        - Scored as: *and, as, at, ~~one~~, said, into, could* = 6 words identified correctly.
- Hesitations with response: Starting to respond but not finishing by 5 seconds and being prompted by pointing to the next word and saying "**What word?**"
    - *Example*: *and, as, at, one, said, into, could*
        - Student says: /and/ /as/ /at/ /ooooonnnnnn/ (hesitates 5 seconds on *one*). Point to *said* and say "**What word?**" /said/ /into/ /could/.
        - Scored as: *and, as, at, ~~one~~, said, into, could* = 6 words identified correctly.
- Reversals: Transposes two or more words.
    - *Example*: *and, as, at, one, said, into, could*
        - Student says: /and/ /as/ /at/ /one/ /into/ /said/ /could/.
        - Scored as: *and, as, at, one, ~~said~~, ~~into~~, could* = 5 words identified correctly.

Special Administration and Scoring Considerations for Word Identification CBM

1. Correction procedure: If the student makes an error, he is not corrected.
2. Skip an entire row: If a student skips an entire row, that row is crossed out and each word is counted as an error.
3. Discontinuation rule: If the student does not get any correct in the first two rows, stop and mark all items as incorrect.
4. If the student finishes in less than 1 minute, note the number of seconds it took to complete the word list and prorate the score. The formula for prorating is:

$$\frac{\text{Total number of correct words}}{\text{Number of seconds it took to finish}} \times 60 = \text{Estimated number of correct words}$$

Example: The student finished the sheet in just 50 seconds and got 35 words correct.

$$\frac{35}{50} \times 60 = 0.7 \times 60 = 42$$

We estimate that the student would have read approximately 42 words correctly in 1 minute had we provided more words and timed the student for the full 1 minute.

5. Elongation of sounds: If the student elongates the sounds in the words and each sound is clearly heard, it is scored as correct.

HOW OFTEN
SHOULD EARLY READING CBM BE ADMINISTERED?

In Chapter 2, we provide additional details on how often and when to administer CBM for the different purposes of universal screening and progress monitoring. Below we provide only an outline for these purposes. We suggest you refer to Chapter 2 for a more in-depth discussion on how often and when to give CBM for these different purposes.

Universal Screening

All students should be screened using grade-level materials three times a year. This typically occurs in fall, winter, and spring. Screening assists in answering some important questions, two of which are:

> "Is this student *at risk* for academic failure by the end of the year?"
> "Is our core instruction meeting the needs of most of our students?"

Progress Monitoring

Only those students who have been identified as *at risk*, meaning they did not score at or above the benchmark score on the universal screening assessment, should be progress monitored at least once a week on instructional-level material and at least once per month on grade-level materials if different from instructional level. An important aspect of progress monitoring is to do it often (i.e., weekly) and consistently (i.e., using CBM materials that are at the same difficulty level). Progress monitoring data assist in answering two very important questions:

> "Is this student benefiting from the instruction she is receiving?"
> "Is this intervention helping the majority of the students who have received it?"

HOW MUCH TIME DOES IT TAKE
TO ADMINISTER AND SCORE EARLY READING CBM?

The time needed to administer and score each student sheet is typically the same for all Early Reading CBM tasks. Once the student is in front of the teacher/examiner, the time it takes to give the directions, have the student respond for 1 minute, and score the sheet is 2–3 minutes total. If you are universally screening and giving three sheets at one time it should take 5–6 minutes total. You will also need to factor in time for the student to move to where the teacher/examiner is, whether that is in the same room or down the hall. Obviously, it makes more sense to go to the students rather than have the students come to the examiner as one way to save time. Another way to save time is to have everything printed out and ready to go with the students' names already indicated on the appropriate forms.

One way to do this is to print labels. Using a system that allows the teacher/examiner to score the assessments online not only saves time needed for scoring and graphing but for the overall organization necessary when testing a lot of students.

READING CBM SCORES

Proficiency Levels or Benchmarks for Early Reading CBM

It is important to have standards for level of performance in order to determine if a student is on track given her current performance as well as predicting how she might perform in the future. These are often referred to as benchmarks. Benchmarks are helpful because they are predictive of later student achievement. Most early reading curriculum-based measures now provide benchmark scores. This is helpful for teachers because it allows them to determine who is on track and who needs additional assistance to be successful at reading. The benchmark scores we provide in Table 3.3 are a sample from various early CBM assessments and align with the measures we highlighted within this chapter. The benchmark scores provide the lowest score we would accept that would indicate a student is *not* at risk for future academic failure.

Norms for Early Reading CBM

Another way to set standards for performance is to compare a student's score to the performance of others in her grade or at her instructional level. However, whenever benchmarks are available those are the data that should be used to make decisions about how well students are performing. Benchmarks are also the preferred metric when writing IEP goals

TABLE 3.3. Example of Benchmarks for Early Literacy CBM Assessments

CBM task	Publisher	K Fall	K Winter	K Spring	1 Fall	1 Winter	1 Spring
Onset Sounds	FastBridge Learning	12	15	—	—	—	—
Phoneme Segmenting[a]	DIBELS	—	20	40	40	—	—
Letter Naming[b]	DIBELS	29	52	62	58	—	—
Letter Sounds	FastBridge Learning	9	29	41	31	43	—
Nonsense Words	FastBridge Learning	—	6	11	9	14	20
Word Identification/ Sight Words	FastBridge Learning	—	6	18	20	48	64

Note. Benchmarks for each assessment are based on specific publisher recommendations. Educators should use only those benchmarks that align with the materials being used.
[a]Benchmarks recommended from Dynamic Measurement Group, Inc. (2010).
[b]Benchmarks recommended from University of Oregon Center on Teaching and Learning (2012).

and objectives, as the score refers to a student being able to reach proficiently by a set point in time. However, we also understand that many people value and appreciate using norms as well. For that reason, we provide norms from FastBridge Learning for onset sounds, phoneme segmenting (referred to as word blending), letter names, letter sounds, nonsense words, and word identification (referred to as sight words) in Appendix A.

HOW DO I USE THE INFORMATION TO WRITE EARLY READING IEP GOALS AND OBJECTIVES?

Here is an example of how Early Reading CBM data can be used to write goals and objectives following the principles outlined in Chapter 2 that focus on time, learner, behavior (e.g., produces sounds, reads), level (kindergarten, first grade), content (e.g., reading), material (LS CBM progress-monitoring material), and criteria (reflecting the norms or benchmarks for that skill, including time and accuracy). We encourage you to review Chapter 2 for further information.

Example of Goal
- Letter Sounds CBM goal
  - In 30 weeks, Lindsay will produce letter sounds from a kindergarten reading sheet of random letters from Letter Sounds CBM progress monitoring material at 35 letter sounds correct in 1 minute with greater than 95% accuracy.

The same principles apply to writing objectives, but one should use a shorter time frame.

Example of Objectives
- Letter Sounds CBM objective
  - In 10 weeks, Lindsay will produce letter sounds from a kindergarten reading sheet of random letters from LS CBM progress-monitoring material at 15 LSC in 1 minute with greater than 95% accuracy.

FREQUENTLY ASKED QUESTIONS ABOUT EARLY READING CBM

1. *What happens if I start the stopwatch and the student starts reading silently?* You should stop the student. Get a different sheet at the same difficulty level, remind him that he needs to read aloud so that you can hear him, and start over, including reading the directions.

2. *If the student is not making good progress, should I lower the goal?* No. The first step should be to determine if the appropariate assessment is being used and if the progress-

monitoring data were collected and graphed correctly. The next step would be to look at the instruction and see if it is appropriate and implemented with fidelity. These steps align with troubleshooting within CBE.

3. *How long do I have to wait to raise the goal if the student is performing better than I thought he would?* After collecting at least six to eight data points, if the student has four *consecutive* data points above the goal line, then it should be raised.

4. *Can I make my own early reading sheets or do I have to purchase them?* We recommend that you purchase them to save time and to ensure that they are all of equivalent difficulty level.

5. *How much training does it typically take to learn how to do Early Reading CBM?* We have found that after practicing with 7 to 10 students, people are typically very good at conducting Early Reading CBM.

6. *Can I change the directions or how I score the sheets/lists?* No. These measures were researched using the standardized procedures we have provided. If the directions or scoring criteria are changed, then the measure is changed, and we do not know what the reliability and validity are.

7. *Do Early Reading CBM measures come in languages other than English?* Yes. Many publishers of Early CBM material have Spanish versions. We have indicated this in Box 3.1 on where to obtain materials.

8. *Can I preteach the letter sounds or the words on the list?* No. This is an assessment and the goal is to determine what skills a student has without help. It is a good thing to teach letter sounds and words, but it is important not to combine the testing and teaching of these skills.

9. *Can I send the CBM sheets home for the student to practice?* No. These are tests and should not be used for practice.

10. *Can I use benchmark scores on CBM to put students in instructional groups?* Yes, if you have students with similar instructional needs. These groups should be flexible and students should be evaluated and regrouped every 6–8 weeks.

11. *Not everyone in my class is on the same instructional level. Should I still give them all the same CBM sheets?* Yes. Because these skills are basic, all students in kindergarten and first grade should be given the same CBM tests. Remember, when you screen, it should always be done on students' grade-level skills.

12. *I only have 20 Letter Sounds or Word Identification CBM sheets, but I need to progress monitor for 35 weeks. Is it OK to use the same sheets again?* Yes. Once you have used all 20, start using them again. The student probably doesn't remember specific items she did 20 weeks ago. This also means that you should not use the sheets as homework or additional practice if you want to use them again.

RESOURCES AND/OR FURTHER READING

Center on Teaching and Learning, University of Oregon (*ctl.uoregon.edu*). Includes instruction and assessment products for literacy and math and online training.

Clemens, N. H., Shapiro, E., Wu, J. Y., Taylor, A. B., & Cadkie, G. L. (2014). Monitoring early first-grade reading progress: A comparison of two measures. *Journal of Learning Disabilities, 47,* 254–270.

Florida Center for Reading Research (*fcrr.org*). Includes student activities for literacy instruction, information about reading assessments, and articles on literacy-related topics.

Fuchs, L. S., Fuchs, D., & Compton, D. L. (2004). Monitoring early reading development in first grade: Word identification fluency versus nonsense word fluency. *Exceptional Children, 71,* 7–21.

Good, R. H., Simmons, D. C., & Smith, S. B. (1998). Effective academic interventions in the United States: Evaluating and enhancing the acquisition of early reading skills. *School Psychology Review, 27*(1), 45–56.

Intervention Central—CBM Warehouse (*www.interventioncentral.org/htmdocs/interventions/cbmwarehouse.shtml*). Includes CBM materials for screening and progress monitoring along with information on using CBM and interpreting results from CBM data.

Iowa Reading Research Center (*www.iowareadingresearch.org*). Includes a collection of web-based literacy resources for families and educators searchable by skill, age, or grade, and common core standards.

IRIS Center, Peabody College, Vanderbilt University (*www.iris.peabody.vanderbilt.edu*). Includes information on evidence-based practices and interventions with a focus on students with disabilities.

Juniper Gardens Children's Project, University of Kansas (*jgcp.ku.edu*). Includes information related to research projects and publications focused on children's developmental and educational experiences to enhance academic and social outcomes.

Kaminski, R. A., & Good R. H. (1996). Toward a technology for assessing early literacy skills. *School Psychology Review, 25,* 215–227.

National Center on Intensive Intervention (*www.intensiveintervention.org*). Includes charts evaluating CBM tools for progress monitoring in academics and behavior, along with webinars and other publications related to assessment and interventions.

Reading Rockets (*www.readingrockets.org*). Includes guides, videos, articles, and other resources focused on supporting students to be successful readers.

Speece, D. L., Mills, C., Ritchey, K. D., & Hillman, E. (2003). Initial evidence that letter fluency tasks are valid indicators of early reading skills. *Journal of Special Education, 36,* 223–233.

Vaughn Gross Center for Reading and Language Arts (*www.Meadowscenter.org*). Includes articles and professional development resources with a focus on struggling readers, English language learners, and students in special education.

CHAPTER 4

How to Conduct Reading CBM

WHY SHOULD I CONDUCT READING CBM?

Many students struggle with reading. Because of this and because it is critical to success in and out of school, it should be assessed often. Reading CBM provides a reliable and valid way to (1) identify if the core instructional program is working, (2) identify students who are at risk for reading failure, (3) identify which students are not making adequate progress given the instruction they are receiving, (4) identify students' instructional level, and (5) identify which students need additional diagnostic evaluation. Over 30 years of research has shown that there is no other assessment that does these things as well as CBM. As mentioned in Chapter 3, most other reading assessments do not provide an account of rate, often referred to as fluency, which allows us to determine how automatic students are at performing a task. Remember, automaticity is important as it demonstrates mastery of skills as well as accounting for unique variance in students' reading ability (Fuchs, Fuchs, Hosp, & Jenkins, 2001).

The two best reasons for conducting Reading CBM are (1) it is easy and time efficient to administer and score and (2) it provides educators with information that can be used to inform instruction at a district, building, grade, classroom, or student level. The CBE process is helpful in determining at what level to intervene. For example, just because a student is having difficulty does not mean the best place to intervene is with that one student if in fact many students are having difficulty. It might make more sense to intervene with a small group, whole class, or grade.

Unlike Early Reading CBM, for which the number of measures available have expanded, Reading CBM still consists of oral passage reading (OPR; reading aloud from a passage for 1 minute) and maze passage reading (i.e., reading a passage silently and restoring every seventh word that has been deleted and replaced with three words).

Each of these assessments provides a different score, but all scores are based on the number of items correct in a set amount of time. This reflects the student's accuracy and fluency on the task. This information provides a database for each student so that appropriate instructional decisions can be made in a timely manner.

Once you have identified which Reading CBM assessments are most appropriate to use, the next step is to gather the materials you will need to conduct CBM. The first assessment we address, OPR (also known as oral reading fluency [ORF] and passage reading fluency [PRF]), is the most commonly used for Reading CBM. We prefer the term *oral passage reading*, as it most accurately reflects the task. The term *fluency* tends to confuse people as it refers to a literacy skill and has instructional implications. If we were to teach fluency, we would have students focus on three things: (1) the correct pace at which you would read a piece of text as it is meant to be read; (2) reading each word accurately within the text it is written; and (3) using the appropriate expression that the text implies. OPR is not a skill one would teach, but rather it can be used as a proxy to measure many skills that are necessary for students to be able to read. The skills students use when reading include decoding, vocabulary, comprehension (accessing prior knowledge), and fluency (pace, accuracy, and expression).

The score for OPR is comprised of the number of words attempted minus the number of errors to provide the number of words read correctly (WRC) within 1 minute. This score provides a robust measure of overall reading competence and is a good predictor of future reading performance.

This chapter will cover the materials needed and the administration and scoring rules for OPR CBM, and we provide the same information for Maze CBM. Maze CBM is actually a better predictor than OPR CBM of future reading performance for students in the higher grades (fourth or higher). In addition, it appears to have slightly better face validity than OPR CBM for its relationship to comprehension (i.e., many people have trouble understanding the relationship between OPR and comprehension, but not the relationship between Maze CBM and comprehension; a reason for this is probably that Maze CBM is more similar to other comprehension measures than OPR CBM). To help you easily find OPR CBM and Maze CBM materials we provide sources in Box 4.1.

OPR CBM

OPR CBM is designed to assess overall reading skills that are also highly predictive of later reading skills.

Materials Needed to Conduct OPR CBM

1. Different but equivalent reading passages (student and teacher/examiner copies).
2. Directions for administering and scoring OPR CBM.
3. A writing utensil and clipboard or computer to enter student responses.
4. A stopwatch or countdown timer that displays seconds.

BOX 4.1. Where to Find Premade Reading CBM Passages (OPR and Maze)

$ indicates there is a cost for the passages and/or graphing program.
⌨ indicates computerized administration available.
✍ indicates data management and graphing available.
S indicates Spanish measures are available.

aimsweb (Pearson) $⌨S

Website: *www.aimsweb.com*

Phone: 866-313-6194

Products: • Oral Passage Reading
            • Maze passages

Dynamic Indicators of Basic Early Literacy Skills (DIBELS)

Website: *www.dibels.org*

Phone: 888-943-1240

Products: • Oral Passage Reading
            • Maze passages

EasyCBM $✍

Website: *www.easycbm.com*

Phone: 800-323-9540

Products: • Oral Passage Reading
            • Multiple Choice Reading Comprehension

Edcheckup $⌨ ✍

Website: *www.edcheckup.com*

Phone: 612-454-0074

Products: • Oral Passage Reading
            • Maze passages

FastBridge Learning $⌨S

Website: *www.fastbridge.org*

Phone: 612-424-3714

Products: • Oral Passage Reading

Intervention Central ✍

Website: *www.interventioncentral.org*

Products: • Oral Passage Reading (premade and create your own)
            • Maze Passages (create your own)

Project AIM (Alternative Identification Models)

Website: *www.glue.umd.edu/%7Edlspeece/cbmreading/index.html*

Phone: 301-405-6514

Products: • Oral Passage Reading

(continued)

System to Enhance Educational Performance (STEEP) $✍S

Website: *www.isteep.com*

Phone: 800-881-9142

Products: • Oral Passage Reading
           • Maze

Vanderbilt University $ (copying, postage, and handling only)

Website: *www.peerassistedlearningstrategies.com*

Phone: 615-343-4782

E-mail: lynn.a.davies@vanderbilt.edu

Products: • Oral Passage Reading

---

5. A quiet testing environment to work with students.
6. An equal-interval graph or a graphing program to plot the data.

OPR CBM Reading Passages

The OPR CBM passages should be different but equivalent in grade level and should include at least 200 words per passage. The reading skills represented should be ones the student is expected to master throughout the entire school year. Typically, the passages are from the end of the school year. While the passages should be different, they should all be of equivalent difficulty (e.g., at the same grade level). It is important that the passages be as close in difficulty as possible. The best way to accomplish this is to purchase generic passages that have been developed specifically for collecting OPR data. For the purposes of discussing the directions, scoring, and additional considerations we will be referring to Shinn (1989). We recommend people look at specific measures they will be using to ensure they follow the administration and scoring rules applicable for that specific measure, as there are variations among publishers.

We recommend administering all universal screening assessments in one testing session to save setup time and for consistency in obtaining an accurate score, but it can occur across consecutive days if needed. If three samples of the same assessment are to be administered, then the median score is used for the final score and can also be placed as the first data point on the student's graph. After that, 20–30 different but equivalent sheets will be used to monitor student progress in reading throughout the year.

OPR CBM must be administered individually. Two copies of each passage will be needed. The student should have a copy of the OPR CBM passage in front of her, and the teacher/examiner should either have a copy of the OPR CBM passage in front of him on the computer screen or a paper copy to write on and a writing utensil, as well as a timer and the directions. See Figures 4.1 and 4.2 for examples of each type of passage. Note that the teacher/examiner's passage (Figure 4.2) has a running word total at the end of each line. This makes scoring much more efficient.

Pack Your Bags Student Copy

"We're going on a trip!" said Dad when we sat down for
breakfast. "We only have two days to get ready. Everyone
will have to help out"

"Where are we going?" asked Sarah.

"We're going to the city," Dad answered.

"What city?" asked Anthony.

"Boston," said Dad. "It will take us about three hours to
drive there by car. There is a lot you can learn about our country's
past in Boston. Now, let's start planning."

Dad gave us each a bag and told us to pack enough clothes
for three days. Since it was summer, we didn't have to worry
about coats and boots. When Dad checked Sarah's bag he said
she should take a dress incase we went someplace fancy.

When he checked my bag he said, "Don't forget your
toothbrush!" He got to Anthony's bag and found it full of toys.
"Anthony, where are your clothes?" He helped him decide
which toys to leave behind so he could fit some clothes in the
bag.

That night, we talked about our trip. "Where will we stay
when we get to Boston?" I asked.

"We'll stay in a hotel right across from Copley Square,"
said Dad.

FIGURE 4.1. Example of student OPR CBM passage. From Edcheckup (2005). Reprinted with permission from Children's Educational Services, Inc., and Edcheckup, LLC.

Directions and Scoring Procedures for OPR CBM

For your convenience, Appendix B includes a reproducible version of the directions and scoring rules for OPR CBM.

Directions for OPR CBM[1]

1. Place the copy of the student passage in front of the student.
2. Place the teacher/examiner copy on the clipboard so the student cannot see it.
3. Say: **"When I say 'Begin,' start reading aloud at the top of the page. Read across the page** (point to the first line of the passage). **Try to read each word. If you come to a word you don't know, I'll tell it to you. Be sure to do your best reading. Do you have any questions? Begin."** (Trigger stopwatch or timer for 1 minute.)

---

[1]Adapted with permission from Shinn (1989).

4. Follow along on the teacher/examiner copy as the student reads and put a slash (/) through any incorrect words.

5. At the end of 1 minute, say **"Thank You"** and mark the last word read with a bracket (]).

Scoring OPR CBM

Submit the results using the online system. Or:

1. Count the total number of items attempted.
2. Count the total number of errors.
3. Calculate rate: Total items attempted – total errors = total correct per minute.
4. Calculate accuracy: Total correct ÷ total items attempted = percent correct.

Pack Your Bags	Examiner Copy
"We're going on a trip!" said Dad when we sat down for	12
breakfast. "We only have two days to get ready. Everyone	22
will have to help out."	27
"Where are we going?" asked Sarah.	33
"We're going to the city," Dad answered.	40
"What city?" asked Anthony.	44
"Boston, said Dad. "It will take us about three hours to	55
drive there by car. There is a lot you can learn about our	68
country's past in Boston. Now, let's start planning."	76
Dad gave us each a bag and told us to pack enough clothes	89
for three days. Since it was summer, we didn't have to worry	101
about coats and boots. When Dad checked Sarah's bag he said	112
she should take a dress incase we went someplace fancy.	123
When he checked my bag he said, "Don't forget your	133
toothbrush!" He got to Anthony's bag and found it full of toys.	145
"Anthony, where are your clothes?" He helped him decide	154
which toys to leave behind so he could fit some clothes in the	167
bag.	168
That night, we talked about our trip. "Where will we stay	179
when we get to Boston?" I asked.	186
"We'll stay in a hotel right across from Copley Square,"	196
said Dad.	198
	Words Correct _____
	Words Incorrect _____

FIGURE 4.2. Example of teacher/examiner OPR CBM passage. Reprinted with permission from Children's Educational Services, Inc., and Edcheckup, LLC.

SCORED AS CORRECT

OPR CBM is scored based on each word being read accurately within the context of the sentence. Having a black-and-white scoring process increases the reliability of scores between students and assists in ensuring the process remains manageable but still provides good data for each student.

- Pronounced correctly: A word must be pronounced correctly, in accordance with the context of the sentence.
  - *Example*: For the sentence *He will read the book*, the word *read* must be pronounced "reed."
    - Student says: "He will *read* the book."
    - Scored as: *He will read the book.* = 5 words read correctly.
    - Student says: "He will *red* the book."
    - Scored as: *He will read the book.* = 4 words read correctly.
- Self-corrections within 3 seconds: Words misread initially but corrected within 3 seconds.
  - *Example*: *The dog licked Kim.*
    - Student says: "The dog *liked* . . . (2 seconds) . . . licked Kim."
    - Scored as: *The dog licked Kim.* = 4 words read correctly.
- Dialect/articulation: Variations in pronunciation explainable by local language norms or speech sound production.
  - *Example*: *I need a pen to sign my name.*
    - Student says: "I need a *pin* to sign my name."
    - Scored as: *I need a pen to sign my name.* = 8 words read correctly.
- Repetitions: Repeating the same word more than once.
  - *Example*: *Bill jumped high.*
    - Student says: "Bill jumped . . . jumped high."
    - Scored as: *Bill jumped high.* = 3 words read correctly.
- Insertions: Adding extra words to the story.
  - *Example*: *The big dog ran home.*
    - Student says: "The big *black* dog ran home."
    - Scored as: *The big dog ran home.* = 5 words read correctly.

SCORED AS ERRORS

All errors are marked with a slash (/) through the word.

- Mispronunciations/word substitutions: When a word is either mispronounced or substituted with another word.
  - *Example*: *The house was big.*
    - Student says: "The *horse* was big."
    - Scored as: The house was big. = 3 words read correctly.

- *Example*: *Mother went to the store.*
  - Student says: "*Mom* went to the store."
  - Scored as: ~~Mother~~ went to the store. = 4 words read correctly.
- Omissions: Words that are not spoken.
  - *Example*: *Juan went to a birthday party.*
    - Student says: "Juan went to a party."
    - Scored as: *Juan went to a ~~birthday~~ party.* = 5 words read correctly.
- Hesitations without response: Not responding for 3 seconds and being prompted by having the word read.
  - *Example*: *Leslie is moving to Miami.*
    - Student says: "Leslie is moving to . . . (3 seconds)" [Provide the word *Miami* and mark it as an error.]
    - Scored as: *Leslie is moving to ~~Miami~~.* = 4 words read correctly.
- Hesitations with response: Starting to respond but not finishing by 3 seconds and being prompted by having the word read.
  - *Example*: *The apple was rotting on one side.*
    - Student says: "The apple was rrrrrooooo (3 seconds) [Provide the word *rotting* and mark it as an error.] on one side."
    - Scored as: *The apple was ~~rotting~~ on one side.* = 6 words read correctly.
- Reversals: Transposing two or more words.
  - *Example*: *The fat cat walked past us.*
    - Student says: "The cat fat walked past us."
    - Scored as: *The ~~fat cat~~ walked past us.* = 4 words read correctly.

Special Administration and Scoring Considerations for OPR CBM

1. Correction procedure: If the student makes an error, she is not corrected. The only time you provide the correct word is if she hesitates for 3 seconds.
2. Skip an entire line: If the student skips a line, you draw a line through it and do *not* count it in the scoring as attempted or errors.
3. Discontinuation rule: If the student reads fewer than 10 words correctly in 1 minute, do not administer additional passages at the same level.
4. Finish before 1 minute: If the student finishes in less than 1 minute, note the number of seconds it took to complete the passage and prorate the score. The formula for prorating is:

$$\frac{\text{Total number of words read correctly}}{\text{Number of seconds to read the passage}} \times 60 = \text{Estimated number of words read correctly in 1 minute}$$

Example: The student finished reading the passage in just 54 seconds and got 44 words correct.

$$\frac{44}{54} \times 60 = 0.815 \times 60 = 49$$

We estimate that the student would have read approximately 49 words correctly in 1 minute had we provided more words and timed her for the full 1 minute.

5. Loses her place: If a student loses her place on the page, point to the items she is on. (Use as often as needed.)

6. Numerals: Numbers are counted as words and must be read correctly within the context of the passage.
   - *Example: August 6, 2003*
     - Student says: "August six, two thousand-three."
     - Scored as: *August 6, 2003* = 3 words read correctly.
     - Student says: "August six, two zero zero three."
     - Scored as: *August 6, 2003* = 2 words read correctly.

7. Hyphenated words: Each morpheme separated by a hyphen(s) is counted as an individual word if it can stand alone.
   - *Son-in-law* = 3 words read correctly.
   - *Forty-five* = 2 words read correctly.
   - *bar-b-que* = 1 word read correctly.
   - *re-evaluate* = 1 word read correctly.

8. Abbreviations: Abbreviations are counted as words and must be read correctly within the context of the sentence (e.g., Mrs., Dr.).
   - *Example: Dr., Mrs., Ms., Mr.*
     - Should be read as: "doctor, missus, miz, mister" = 1 word read correctly each.
     - *Not* "D-R, M-R-S, M-S, M-R." = 0 words read correctly each.

MAZE CBM

Maze CBM is designed to assess overall reading skills, similarly to OPR CBM. Research has indicated that once students master the foundational skills and are able to read at an appropriate rate with high accuracy, Maze performs as a better proxy and has a higher correlation with comprehension. This typically occurs after third grade. We have included an example of two sets of administration directions from two different sources. Just as with OPR CBM, it is important to use the same set of directions each time within a school or district if the data will be used to make comparisons across classrooms, grades, or schools. Changing the directions can change how the student performs on the task and, therefore, should be avoided.

Materials Needed to Conduct Maze CBM

1. Different but equivalent Maze passages (student and teacher/examiner copies).
2. Directions for administering and scoring Maze CBM.
3. A writing utensil and clipboard or computer for student to enter their responses.
4. A stopwatch or countdown timer that displays seconds.
5. A quiet testing environment to work with students.
6. An equal-interval graph or a graphing program to plot the data.

Maze Reading Passages

The reading passages should be different but equivalent in level of difficulty and should include at least 300 words and 42 deleted words (with three replacement words each). The reading skills should represent the skills the student is expected to master by the end of the school year. While the passages should be different, they should all be of equivalent difficulty. The best way to accomplish this is to purchase generic passages that have been developed specifically for this purpose.

We recommend administering all universal screening assessments in one testing session to save setup time and for consistency in obtaining an accurate score, but it can occur across consecutive days if needed. If three samples of the CBM task are to be administered, then the median score is used for the final score and can also be placed as the first data point on the student's graph. After that, 20–30 different but equivalent passages will be used to monitor student progress in reading throughout the year.

Maze passages can be administered to a group. The students should each have a copy of the Maze CBM passage in front of them, and the teacher/examiner should have a copy of the administration directions and a timer. To score the passages, the teacher/examiner will also need the examiner copy of the Maze passage with the answers (see Figures 4.3 and 4.4 for an example of each) and a writing utensil. Scoring can be facilitated by making a transparency of a correctly scored passage. This transparency can then be placed over the student's work for rapid error recognition.

Name _____   Date _____

The Visitor   Student Copy

Tap, tap, tap. I was reading a book. But (**I, top, bit**) kept hearing a noise at the (**red, eat, window**). Tap, tap. I began reading again. (**Clunk, Top, Ball**) scrape, tap, tap. I looked out (**stick, of, sit**) the window. It was dark outside. (**I, Did, A**) couldn't see anything. I looked back (**tick, pit, at**) my book. It was hard to (**so, find, and**) my place. I found it and (**it, began, tree**) to read. I heard the noise (**up, again, into**). This time I was not going (**bad, to, an**) stop reading. I didn't want to (**hit, tip, lose**) my place again.

Clunk, scrape, scrape. (**I, Dig, Ran**) had to look up again. I (**lip, nap, was**) mad. I knew I had lost (**stop, my, jump**) place. I just had to find (**map, out, tan**) what was making that noise on (**din, the, still**) window. I walked to the door. (**I, At, Six**) turned on the outside light. Tap, (**scrape, hill, back**). I stepped outside to look at (**blue, the, what**) window. There it was—a big (**June, walk, sit**) bug. It kept flying against the (**in, who, window**) again and again. Now I knew (**rip, too, I**) had a visitor. I didn't need (**sip, to, live**) stop to check it out again, (**you, ping, so**) I just went back to my (**its, up, reading**).

Correct _____

Incorrect _____

FIGURE 4.3. Example of student Maze CBM passage. Reprinted with permission from Children's Educational Services, Inc., and Edcheckup, LLC.

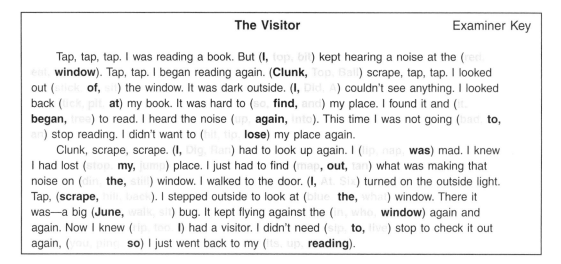

FIGURE 4.4. Example of teacher/examiner Maze CBM passage. Reprinted with permission from Children's Educational Services, Inc., and Edcheckup, LLC.

Directions and Scoring Procedures for Maze CBM

We provide two sets of administration directions for Maze CBM to reflect how it would be conducted if (1) you were using practice items, or (2) you were providing the directions without practice items. For your convenience, Appendix B includes a reproducible version of the directions and scoring rules for Maze CBM.

Directions for Maze CBM with Practice Items[2]

1. Place a copy of the student passage with the practice items in front of each student (see Figure 4.5 for an example of the practice items).
2. Say: *"Today I want you to read a short story. The story you will read has some places where you will need to choose the correct word. Read the story. When you come to three words in dark print, choose the word that belongs in the sentence.*

    "We will do some examples. Look at the first page. Read the sentence. The sentence says: 'Bill threw the ball to Jane. Jane caught the (dog, bat, ball).' *Which one of the three words belongs in the sentence?"*
3. After the students respond, say: *"The word 'ball' belongs in the sentence 'Bill threw the ball to Jane. Jane caught the ball.' Circle the word 'ball.'"*
4. *"Now let's try sentence number 2. Read the sentence. The sentence says: 'Tom said, "Now you* (jump, throw, talk) *the ball to me."' Which of the three words belongs in the sentence?"*
5. After the students respond, say: *"The word 'throw' belongs in the sentence 'Now you throw the ball to me.' Circle the word 'throw.'"*
6. Place a copy of the student passage in front of each student face down.

---

[2]Adapted with permission from Edcheckup (2005).

Name _____ Date _____

Maze Procedure
Student Practice Examples

1. Bill threw the ball to Jane. Jane caught the (**dog, bat, ball**).

2. Tom said, "Now you (**jump, throw, talk**) the ball to me."

FIGURE 4.5. Maze CBM practice item. Reprinted with permission from Children's Educational Services, Inc., and Edcheckup, LLC.

7. Say: *"Now you are going to do the same thing by yourself. You will read a story for 1 minute. When I say 'Stop,' stop reading. Do not begin reading until I tell you to start. Whenever you come to three words that are in dark print, circle the word that belongs in the sentence.*

    "Choose a word even if you're not sure of the answer. At the end of 1 minute, I will say 'Stop.' If you finish early, check your answers. Do not go on to the next page. You may turn your paper over and begin when I say 'Start.' Are there any questions?

    "Remember to do the best you can. Pick up your pencils. Ready? Start." (*Trigger stopwatch or timer for 1 minute.*)

8. Walk around the room to monitor students and make sure they are only circling one word per set and not skipping around the page.

9. At the end of 1 minute, say: *"Stop. Put your pencils down."*

10. Separately administer two more passages using the following directions.

11. Say: *"Now you will do the same thing with another story. Remember to choose the word that belongs in the sentence. Choose a word even if you're not sure of the answer. You may begin when I tell you to."* (*Trigger stopwatch or timer for 1 minute.*)

12. At the end of 1 minute, say: *"Stop. Put your pencils down."*

13. Collect all the students' sheets.

Directions for Maze CBM without Practice Items[3]

1. Place a copy of the student passage in front of each student face down. (It is helpful to have the student's name already on the sheet before starting.)

2. Say: *"When I say 'Begin,' turn to the first story and start reading silently. When you come to a group of three words, circle the one word that makes the most sense. Work as quickly as you can without making mistakes. If you finish the page, turn the page and keep working until I say 'Stop' or you are all done. Do you have any questions? Begin."* (*Trigger stopwatch or timer for 3 minutes.*)

3. Walk around the room to monitor students and make sure they are only circling one word per set and not skipping around the page.

---

[3]Adapted with permission from aimsweb (Shinn & Shinn, 2002b).

4. At the end of 3 minutes, say: *"Stop. Put your pencil down and turn your sheet over."*
5. Collect all the students' sheets.

Scoring Maze CBM

Submit the results using the online system. Or:

1. Count the total number of responses attempted in 3 minutes, or whatever time period is specified by for the materials you are using (other common time limits are 1 minute or 2½ minutes).
2. Count the total number of errors.
3. Calculate rate: Total items attempted – total errors = total correct per (1–3 minutes).
4. Calculate accuracy: total correct ÷ total items attempted = percent correct.

SCORED AS CORRECT

Maze CBM is scored based on the student picking the correct word to restore the meaning to the sentence. The student must circle or underline his choice.

- Answered correctly: The correct word is circled or underlined.
  - *Example*: The big dog (**slept,** **ran,** **can**) fast.
    - Student responds: The big dog (**slept,** **ran**, **can**) fast.
    - Scored as: Correct.

SCORED AS ERRORS

All errors are marked by putting a slash (∕) through the correct choice if the incorrect word is circled, underlined, or left blank.

- *Example*: The (**turtle, boy, pulls**) has a little tail.
  - Student responds: The (**turtle,** **boy,** **pulls**) has a little tail.
  - Scored as: The (**turtle,** **boy,** **pulls**) has a little tail. = incorrect.
  - Student responds: The (**turtle,** **boy,** **pulls**) has a little tail.
  - Scored as: The (**turtle,** **boy,** **pulls**) has a little tail. = incorrect.
  - Student responds: The (**turtle,** **boy,** **pulls**) has a little tail.
  - Scored as: The (**turtle,** **boy,** **pulls**) has a little tail. = incorrect.

Special Administration and Scoring Considerations for Maze CBM

1. Correction procedure: If the student makes an error, she is not corrected. The only time an answer is provided is if the student makes an error on a practice item.
2. Skip an entire line: Any items skipped are counted as errors.

3. Discontinuation rule: As this assessment is given in a group format there is no discontinuation rule.

4. Finish before time is up: If the student finishes before 3 minutes, write the number of minutes and seconds on the student's sheet and prorate her score. The formula for prorating is:

$$\text{Step 1:} \quad \frac{\text{Total number of seconds}}{\text{Number of correct answers}} = \text{Calculated value}$$

$$\text{Step 2:} \quad \frac{\text{Total number of seconds in minutes}}{\text{Calculated value}} = \text{Estimated total correct}$$

Example: The student finished the Maze passage in 2 minutes and 30 seconds (150 seconds) and got 40 correct.

$$\text{Step 1:} \quad \frac{150}{40} = 3.75$$

$$\text{Step 2:} \quad \frac{180}{3.75} = 48 \text{ estimated total correct}$$

We estimate that the student would have correctly restored 48 words in 3 minutes had we provided more words and timed the student for the full 3 minutes. (*Note:* 180 is the total number of seconds in 3 minutes. If you need to prorate for a scale that uses a different time interval, convert the number of minutes to seconds.)

5. Stop scoring: If three consecutive responses are incorrect, then you do not count or score any of the responses following the three consecutive incorrect.

6. Directions for group versus individual administration: The same directions are used for group and/or individual administration.

HOW OFTEN SHOULD OPR CBM AND MAZE CBM BE ADMINISTERED?

Knowing *when* to give a CBM measure depends on the purpose for which you are giving it. Chapter 2 provides an overview of purposes for universal screening and progress monitoring. Below we give information for each but would recommend referring back to Chapter 2 for more details.

Universal Screening

All students should be screened using grade-level materials three times a year. This typically occurs in fall, winter, and spring. Universal screening data assist in answering some important questions, two of which are:

"Is this student *at risk* for academic failure by the end of the year?"

"Is our core instruction meeting the needs of most of our students?"

Progress Monitoring

Only those students who have been identified as *at risk,* meaning they did not score at or above the benchmark score on the universal screening assessment, should be progress monitored at least once a week on instructional level material and at least once per month on grade-level materials if different from instructional level. An important aspect of progress monitoring is to do it often (i.e., weekly) and consistently (i.e., using CBM materials that are at the same difficulty level). Progress monitoring data assist in answering two very important questions:

"Is this student benefiting from the instruction he is receiving?"

"Is this intervention helping the majority of the students who have received it?"

HOW MUCH TIME DOES IT TAKE TO ADMINISTER AND SCORE READING CBM?

The time needed to score each student passage varies slightly for OPR CBM and Maze CBM. For OPR CBM, once the student is in front of the teacher/examiner, the time it takes to give the directions, have the student read for 1 minute, and score the passage is 2–3 minutes total. If you are universally screening and giving three passages at one time, it should take 5–6 minutes total. You will also need to factor in time for the student to move to where the teacher/examiner is, whether that is in the same room or down the hall. Obviously, it makes more sense to go to the students rather than have the students come to the examiner as one way to save time. Another way to save time is to have everything printed out and ready to go with the students' names already indicated on the appropriate forms. One way to do this is to print labels. Using a system that allows the teacher/examiner to score the assessments online not only saves time needed for scoring and graphing but for the overall organization necessary when testing a lot of students.

For Maze CBM, once the student is in front of the teacher/examiner, the time it takes to give the directions, have the student read for 3 minutes, and score the passage is 4–5 minutes total. If you are universally screening and giving three passages at one time, it should take 12–15 minutes total. While students in older grades may make more restorations, this should not increase the time needed to score the passage. One way to save time is to have an overlay with the correct answers on it that the teacher/examiner can place over the Maze passage. All the teacher/examiner would have to do is count the number of errors and subtract this from the total attempted. Remember that OPR CBM must be given individually, but that Maze CBM can be given to a whole class. So the time to administer it to a group would be the same, but you would need to add 20–30 seconds to score all of your student's passages.

READING CBM SCORES

Proficiency Levels or Benchmarks for Reading CBM

It is important to have standards for level of performance in order to determine if a student is on track given his current performance as well as predicting how he might perform in the future. These are often referred to as benchmarks. Benchmarks are helpful because they are predictive of later student achievement. Most CBM reading measures now provide benchmark scores. This is helpful for teachers because it allows them to determine who is on track and who needs additional assistance to be successful at reading. Table 4.1 has benchmark scores for OPR from the DIBELS website and Table 4.2 has benchmark scores for Maze/Daze from the DIBELS website. The benchmark scores provide the lowest score we would accept that would indicate a student is *not* at risk for future academic failure.

Norms for Reading CBM

Another way to set standards for performance is to compare a student's score to the performance of others in her grade or at her instructional level. However, whenever benchmarks are available those are the data that should be used to make decisions about how well students are performing. Benchmarks are also the preferred metric when writing IEP Goals and Objectives as the score refers to a student being able to reach proficiency by a set point in time. However, we also understand that many people value and appreciate using norms as well. For that reason, we provide norms for both OPR and Maze in Appendix A.

HOW DO I USE THE INFORMATION TO WRITE READING IEP GOALS AND OBJECTIVES?

Writing goals and objectives is a helpful way to define the behavior of interest and how it will be measured in order to be able to make decisions about a student's learning. Chapter 2 provides the seven steps needed to write a good goal or objective. The seven steps include:

TABLE 4.1. Benchmarks for ORP CBM: Words Read Correctly (WRC)

	DIBELS (2010)		
Grade	Fall (WRC)	Winter (WRC)	Spring (WRC)
1	—	23	47
2	52	72	87
3	70	86	100
4	90	103	115
5	111	120	130
6	107	109	120

TABLE 4.2. Benchmarks for Maze/Daze CBM: Words Correctly Restored (WCR)

	DIBELS (2010)		
Grade	Fall (WCR)	Winter (WCR)	Spring (WCR)
1	—	—	—
2	—	—	—
3	8	11	19
4	15	17	24
5	18	20	24
6	18	19	21

time, learner, behavior, level, content, material, and criteria. Here, we will provide only an example for OPR and Maze CBM, but we encourage you to look at Chapter 2 for further information.

Example of Goals
- OPR goal
  - In one year, Edgar will read aloud a second-grade passage from OPR CBM progress monitoring material at 90 WRC in 1 minute with greater than 95% accuracy.
- Maze goal
  - In 30 weeks, Devin will correctly restore missing words on a fourth-grade Maze passage from Maze CBM progress-monitoring material at 20 WCR in 3 minutes with greater than 95% accuracy.

The same principles apply to writing objectives, but one should use a shorter time frame.

Example of Objectives
- OPR objective
  - In 10 weeks, Edgar will read aloud a second-grade passage from OPR CBM progress-monitoring material at 50 WRC in 1 minute with greater than 95% accuracy.
- Maze objective
  - In 10 weeks, Devin will correctly restore missing words on a fourth-grade Maze passage from Maze CBM progress-monitoring material at 8 WCR in 3 minutes with greater than 95% accuracy.

FREQUENTLY ASKED QUESTIONS ABOUT READING CBM

1. *For OPR CBM, should I have students read the title on the page or should I read it to them?* This depends on whether this is part of the standard administration for the set of passages you are using. Some publishers include reading the title in the directions while many others do not. You should *only* read the title when it is part of the standardized instructions.

2. *For OPR CBM, what happens if I start the stopwatch and the student starts reading silently?* You should stop the student, remind her that she needs to read aloud so that you can hear her, and start over, including reading the directions.

3. *For OPR CBM, what if the student does not read the first word in 3 seconds?* You should say the word, put a slash through it, and continue to have the student read, keeping the timer going all along.

4. *If the student is not making good progress, should I lower the goal?* No. You should refer to the troubleshooting chapter of *The ABCs of Curriculum-Based Evaluation*. This

provides detailed steps for what to do if the student is *not* making progress. It might be a problem with the assessment, graphing of the data, intensity of instruction, or focus of the instruction. Lowering the goal will not increase the likelihood that the student will learn the skill and should therefore be avoided at all costs.

5. ***How long do I have to wait to raise the goal if the student is performing better than I thought she would?*** If the student has hit the benchmark for the end of that year, then you should go ahead and raise the goal. Another rule of thumb is that after collecting at least six to eight data points, if the student has four *consecutive* data points above the goal line, then it should be raised.

6. ***Can I make my own OPR CBM passages, or do I have to purchase them?*** We strongly recommend that you purchase them to save time and to ensure that they are all of equivalent difficulty level.

7. ***How much training does it typically take to learn how to do OPR and Maze CBM?*** We have found that after practicing with 7 to 10 students, people are typically very good at conducting CBM.

8. ***Can I change the directions or how I score the passages?*** No. These measures were researched using the standardized procedures we have provided. If the directions or scoring criteria are changed, then the measure is changed, and we do not know what the reliability and validity are.

9. ***Do OPR CBM or Maze CBM passages come in languages other than English?*** Yes. Many publishers of CBM passages have Spanish versions (OPR more so than Maze). We have indicated this in Box 4. 1 on where to obtain materials.

10. ***Can I use benchmark scores on OPR CBM to put students in instructional groups?*** Yes, if you have students with similar instructional needs. These groups should be flexible, and students should be evaluated and regrouped every 6–8 weeks.

11. ***Not everyone in my class is on the same instructional level. Should I still give them all the same OPR CBM or Maze CBM passages?*** All students should be screened on their grade level; however, students should be progress monitored on their instructional level—especially if they are receiving instruction on that level. We recommend using both grade- and instructional-level materials for progress monitoring. The weekly progress monitoring would be done using instructional level and an additional monthly progress-monitoring data point would be collected using grade-level material.

12. ***What should I do with the scored passages?*** This information can be kept in a portfolio along with the graphed data to demonstrate progress over the year.

13. ***I only have 20 OPR CBM or Maze CBM passages, but I need to progress monitor for 35 weeks. Is it OK to use the same passages again?*** Yes. Once you have used all 20, start using them again. The student probably doesn't remember specific passages she read 20 weeks ago. This also means that you should not use the passages as homework or additional practice if you want to use them again.

RESOURCES AND/OR FURTHER READING

Bean, R. M., & Lane, S. (1990). Implementing curriculum-based measures of reading in an adult literacy program. *Remedial and Special Education, 11*(5), 39–46.

Bradley-Klug, K. L., Shapiro, E. S., Lutz, J., & DuPaul, G. J. (1998). Evaluation of oral reading rate as a curriculum-based measure within a literature-based curriculum. *Journal of School Psychology, 36*, 183–197.

Center on Teaching and Learning, University of Oregon (*ctl.uoregon.edu*). Includes instruction and assessment products for literacy and math and online training.

Christ, T. J., White, M. J., Ardoin, S. P., & Eckert, T. L. (2013). Curriculum based measurement of reading: Consistency and validity across best, fastest, and question reading conditions. *School Psychology Review, 42*, 415–436.

Florida Center for Reading Research (*fcrr.org*). Includes student activities for literacy instruction, information about reading assessments, and articles on literacy-related topics.

Fuchs, L. S., Fuchs, D., Hosp, M. K., & Hamlett, C. L. (2003). The potential for diagnostic analysis with curriculum-based measurement. *Assessment for Effective Intervention, 28*(3/4), 13–22.

Hintze, J. M., Daly, E. J., & Shapiro, E. S. (1998). An investigation of the effects of passage difficulty level on outcomes of oral reading fluency progress monitoring. *School Psychology Review, 27*, 433–445.

Intervention Central—CBM Warehouse (*www.interventioncentral.org/htmdocs/interventions/cbmwarehouse.shtml*). Includes CBM materials for screening and progress monitoring along with information on using CBM and interpreting results from CBM data.

Iowa Reading Research Center (*www.iowareadingresearch.org*). Includes a collection of web-based literacy resources for families and educators searchable by skill, age or grade, and standards.

IRIS Center, Peabody College, Vanderbilt University (*www.iris.peabody.vanderbilt.edu*). Includes information on evidence-based practices and interventions with a focus on students with disabilities.

Petscher, Y., Cummings, K. D., Biancarosa, G., & Fien, H. (2013). Advanced (Measurement) applications of curriculum-based measurement in reading. *Assessment for Effective Intervention, 38*, 71–75.

Reading Rockets (*www.readingrockets.org*). Includes guides, videos, articles, and other resources focused on supporting students to be successful readers.

Scott, V. G., & Weishaar, M. K. (2003). Curriculum-based measurement for reading progress. *Intervention in School and Clinic, 38*, 153–159.

Shinn, M. R., & Shinn, M. M. (2002). *AIMSweb training workbook: Administration and scoring of reading curriculum-based measurement (R-CBM) for use in general outcome measurement.* Eden Prairie, MN: Edformation.

Vaughn Gross Center for Reading and Language Arts (*www.Meadowscenter.org*). Includes articles and professional development resources with a focus on struggling readers, English language learners, and students in special education.

CHAPTER 5

How to Conduct Spelling CBM

WHY SHOULD I CONDUCT SPELLING CBM?

Spelling is an important skill for writing and evaluating that also provides information about a student's decoding. Good spellers are always good at decoding and reading words, but the reverse is not always true; a poor speller can be a good decoder or word reader or a poor decoder or word reader. Spelling CBM assesses students' ability to generalize learned spelling rules in novel tasks in addition to the number of words students can spell correctly. Research indicates a strong relation between a student's ability to decode and spell, making curriculum-based measures for spelling and decoding an important part of assessing key literacy skills (Robbins, Hosp, Hosp, & Flynn, 2010).

Spelling CBM is a short, sensitive measure of spelling achievement. It can serve as an alternative to traditional weekly spelling tests, which often cannot distinguish between students' actual spelling skill and their ability to memorize or copy words (Loeffler, 2005). It has been field tested for more than 30 years and has been used successfully with general education students (Fuchs, Fuchs, Hamlett, Walz, & Germann, 1993) and students with disabilities (Fuchs, Fuchs, & Hamlett, 1989). As with all other CBM tasks, the information obtained provides a database for each student so that appropriate instructional decisions can be made in a timely manner.

MATERIALS NEEDED TO CONDUCT SPELLING CBM

1. Different but equivalent grade-level spelling lists.
2. Directions for administering and scoring Spelling CBM.
3. Lined paper and writing utensils for student responses.
4. A stopwatch or countdown timer that displays seconds.
5. A quiet testing environment to work with students.
6. An equal-interval graph or a graphing program to plot the data.

SPELLING CBM LISTS

The spelling lists should have different words, include the same number of total letters, be equivalent in grade level, and include 12 words for first and second grade and 17 words for third grade and above. The lists are skills-based measures, meaning that they are composed of items/words selected from across the whole year's spelling curriculum. There are some programs that have already created grade-level spelling lists with equal numbers of correct letter sequences (which makes scoring much faster). These commercial programs typically provide 20–40 alternate forms representing the yearlong curriculum. A source for obtaining spelling lists is provided in Box 5.1.

Purchasing premade lists may not be an option in some situations, but teachers can create their own grade-level spelling lists. Lists must be similar in the number of words and correct letter sequences (CLS). The words should be sampled equally from spelling lists found throughout the yearlong curriculum. To obtain similar levels of CLS, there should be the same number of words of each length (three-letter, four-letter, etc.) in each list. Although specific CLS data do not exist for each grade level, the following can be used as guidelines: first- and second-grade lists should have 55–70 CLS and upper-level lists should have 125–155 CLS.

Just like the other curriculum-based measures, the first time Spelling CBM is administered three equivalent spelling lists should be used, whether you are going to be conducting universal screening or progress monitoring. This should be conducted in one testing session, but it can occur across consecutive days if needed. We recommend doing it in one session to save setup time and obtain a more accurate score. The median score of these three samples will be used to provide the first data point on the student's graph. After that, 20–30 different but equivalent lists will be used to monitor student progress in spelling throughout the year.

Spelling CBM can be administered individually or to a group. The spelling lists will be needed along with the directions and a timer. The student(s) should have lined paper and a pencil or pen. It may be helpful to give each student a spiral notebook for his responses. This allows teachers and students to see progress over time as well as provide a record of student responses. It is also helpful in situations where the measure is given to all students each week even though just a few are being progress monitored. See Figures 5.1 and 5.2 for examples of a spelling list and a scored spelling list.

BOX 5.1. Where to Find Premade Spelling CBM Lists

$ indicates there is a cost for the sheets or lists and/or graphing program.
🖥 indicates computerized administration available.
✍ indicates data management and graphing available.
S indicates Spanish measures are available.

aimsweb (Pearson) $✍

Website: *www.aimsweb.com*

Phone: 866-313-6194

Products: • Spelling

aimsweb® Standard Spelling Progress Monitor Assessment List #4 (3rd Grade)

Given By: _____   Date Given: __ / __ / __

ID	Word	CLS	CCLS
1	tape	5	5
2	supplier	9	14
3	jelly	6	20
4	rooster	8	28
5	cricket	8	36
6	sheriff	8	44
7	house	6	50
8	waste Don't waste good food.	6	56
9	wear What are you going to wear?	5	61
10	away	5	66
11	led She led the class.	4	70
12	ear	4	74
13	woolen	7	81
14	obeyed	7	88
15	onto	5	93
16	wagging	8	101
17	watermelon	11	112
	Total CLS	**112**	

Note. CCLS = Cumulative CLS.

FIGURE 5.1. Example of teacher/examiner Spelling CBM list. From aimsweb (2003). Reprinted with permission from Edformation, Inc.

DIRECTIONS AND SCORING PROCEDURES FOR SPELLING CBM

For your convenience, Appendix B includes a reproducible version of the directions and scoring rules for Spelling CBM.

Directions for Spelling CBM[1]

1. Select an appropriate grade-level spelling list.
2. Have students number their papers from 1 to 12 for first and second graders or 1 to 17 for third grade and up.
3. Say: *"I am going to read some words to you. I want you to write the words on the sheet in front of you. Write the first word on the first line, the second word on the second line, and so on. I'll give you 10 seconds [7 seconds for grade 3 and up] to spell each word.*

---

[1]Adapted with permission from Shinn (1989).

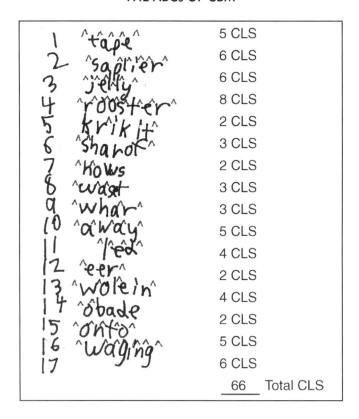

FIGURE 5.2. Example of student Spelling CBM list scored.

When I say the next word, try to write it, even if you haven't finished the last one. Are there any questions?"

4. Say the first word and trigger stopwatch or timer for 2 minutes.
5. Say each word twice. Use homonyms in a sentence.
6. Say a new word every 10 seconds (grades 1 and 2) or 7 seconds (grade 3 and up).
7. At the end of 2 minutes, say: *"Thank you. Put your pencils down."*

Scoring Spelling CBM

Spelling CBM can be scored for CLS and words spelled correctly (WSC). CLS is the total number of pairs of letters that are in the correct sequence; WSC is the total number of words spelled correctly.

1. Count the total number of correct letter sequences to obtain the CLS score.
2. Count the total number of words spelled correctly to obtain the WSC score.

CLS requires more time to score but also offers a more sensitive measure to gauge student improvement. CLS can provide diagnostic information, assess the effectiveness of spelling instruction, and monitor students' progress. A correct letter sequence includes the beginning space to the first letter, letter to letter, a letter to punctuation, punctuation to a letter, and an end letter to a space. CLS is scored using an upper caret (^) to identify each correct sequence. Nothing is used to identify incorrect letter sequences. The CLS for each word is equal to the number of letters in the word plus one, except when punctuation is used; then it is the number of letters in the word plus two.

WSC is easier to score. Each correctly spelled word or its corresponding number is circled, and the total number of circled words is the WSC. WSC is currently used in many spelling programs as an indicator of general spelling skill.

Comparison between WSC and CLS

Example: Five dictated words, scoring for WSC and CLS, and possible CLS

Dictated Words	Student Response	WSC	CLS	Possible CLS
heel	1. ^h^el^	0	3	5 ^h^e^e^l^
wise	2. ^w^ize^	0	3	5 ^w^i^s^e^
don't	3. ^d^o^nt^	0	4	6 ^d^o^n^'^t^
speak	4. ^s^p^e^a^k^	1	6	6 ^s^p^e^a^k^
dinner	5. ^d^i^n^n^e^r^	1	7	7 ^d^i^n^n^e^r^

This example demonstrates how CLS is more sensitive to student improvement than WSC. For WSC, the student got 2 of 5 words correct, which is 40% correct. For CLS, the student got 23 of 29 letter sequences correct, which is 79% correct.

With WSC, the student gets the same credit (0) when spelling *heel* if he writes "xxzz" or "hel." Obviously one is closer to being correct than the other. Using CLS gives the teacher, student, and parent a better idea of *how* close the student is to learning spelling patterns and getting the answer correct.

Scoring Correct Letter Sequences (CLS)

- CLS is the number of correct sequences related to spelling, the space before and after the word, and the letter to punctuation (before and after). When scoring CLS, the scorer places a caret (^) to indicate each correct sequence.
  - *Example*: Dictated word *chair*
    - Student writes: chair
    - Scored as: ^c^h^a^i^r^ = 6 correct letter sequences.
    - Student writes: chars
    - Scored as: ^c^h^a r s = 3 correct letter sequences.
- Compound words: Words need to stay together without a space.
  - *Example*: Dictated word *downhill*
    - Student writes: downhill
    - Scored as: ^d^o^w^n^h^i^l^l^ = 9 correct letter sequences.
    - Student writes: down hill
    - Scored as: ^d^o^w^n h^i^l^l^ = 8 correct letter sequences.

- Apostrophe: The spaces before and after an apostrophe are counted.
  - *Example*: Dictated word *o'clock*
    - Student writes: o'clock
    - Scored as: ^o^'^c^l^o^c^k^ = 8 correct letter sequences.
    - Student writes: oclock
    - Scored as: ^o c^l^o^c^k^ = 6 correct letter sequences.
- Hyphens: The spaces before and after a hyphen are counted.
  - *Example*: Dictated word *sister-in-law*
    - Student writes: sister-in-law
    - Scored as: ^s^i^s^t^e^r^-^i^n^-^l^a^w^ = 14 correct letter sequences.
    - Student writes: sister in law
    - Scored as: ^s^i^s^t^e^r i^n l^a^w^ = 10 correct letter sequences.
- Capitalization: A word that should be capitalized must begin with a capital letter.
  - *Example*: Dictated word *April*
    - Student writes: April
    - Scored as: ^A^p^r^i^l^ = 6 correct letter sequences.
    - Student writes: april
    - Scored as: a p^r^i^l^ = 4 correct letter sequences.
- Repeated letters in sequence: Words with letters that are repeated in sequence are scored the same as if each letter were different.
  - *Example*: Dictated word *bloom*
    - Student writes: bloom
    - Scored as: ^b^l^o^o^m^ = 6 correct letter sequences.
    - Student writes: blom
    - Scored as: ^b^l^o m^ = 4 correct letter sequences.
    - or
    - Scored as: ^b^l o^m^ = 4 correct letter sequences.
- Additional letters: Additional letters are not counted twice.
  - *Example*: Dictated word *correct*
    - Student writes: correct
    - Scored as: ^c^o^r^r^e^c^t^ = 8 correct letter sequences.
    - Student writes: corrrect
    - Scored as: ^c^o^r r r^e^c^t^ = 7 correct letter sequences.
- Insertions: Extra letters at the beginning and end are not counted.
  - *Example*: Dictated word *phone*
    - Student writes: phone
    - Scored as: ^p^h^o^n^e^ = 6 correct letter sequences.
    - Student writes: fphone
    - Scored as: fp^h^o^n^e^ = 5 correct letter sequences.
    - Student writes: phoney
    - Scored as: ^p^h^o^n^e y = 5 correct letter sequences.

Special Administration and Scoring Considerations for Spelling CBM

1. Correction procedure: If the student makes an error, he is not corrected.
2. Skip an item: If a student skips an item it is counted as incorrect. Say **"Try to spell each word."**
3. Discontinuation rule: There is no discontinuation rule for Spelling CBM.
4. Clear pronunciation of words: It is vital that each word be pronounced clearly and at an audible level.
5. Using prompts: Use a prompt for younger students to keep them on the right number every four to five words. Say, for example, **"Number 5 is . . .** (*insert word*)."

HOW OFTEN SHOULD SPELLING CBM BE ADMINISTERED?

In Chapter 2, we provide additional details on how often and when to administer CBM for the different purposes of universal screening and progress monitoring. Below we provide an outline for universal screening and progress monitoring for Spelling CBM. We suggest you refer to Chapter 2 for a more in-depth discussion on how often and when to give CBM for these different purposes.

Universal Screening

All students should be screened using grade level materials three times a year. This typically occurs in fall, winter, and spring. Universal screening data assist in answering some important questions, two of which are:

"Is this student *at risk* for academic failure by the end of the year?"
"Is our core instruction meeting the needs of most of our students?"

Progress Monitoring

Only those students who have been identified as *at risk*, meaning they did not score at or above the benchmark score on the universal screening assessment, should be progress monitored at least once a week on instructional level material and at least once per month on grade-level materials if different from instructional level. An important aspect of progress monitoring is to do it often (i.e., weekly) and consistently (i.e., using CBM materials that are at the same difficulty level). Progress monitoring data assist in answering two very important questions:

"Is this student benefiting from the instruction she is receiving?"
"Is this intervention helping the majority of the students who have received it?"

HOW MUCH TIME DOES IT TAKE
TO ADMINISTER AND SCORE SPELLING CBM?

The time needed to score each student list will depend on the proficiency of the speller, the grade level, and the experience of the scorer. Whether you are giving a test to a class of 25 or an individual student, the time is still 2 minutes for the test itself plus the time for you to get the student(s) ready and collect the sheets. We would estimate that once the students are familiar with the process, it should take about 5 minutes to administer the test.

Knowing the number of CLS for each word and for the total list will assist in scoring. First, it will not be necessary to count the CLS for each word if they are all spelled correctly. Second, if the student misses only a few CLS, you can subtract the difference from the total CLS as opposed to adding the CLS for each word. Third, it may be easier to use a felt-tip pen and make dots instead of carets; however, this should only be used after you have become proficient at scoring Spelling CBM. We estimate that it would take no longer than 10–15 seconds to score WSC and 30 seconds to score CLS if the total CLS is already known.

SPELLING CBM SCORES

It is important to know what the expected level of performance is throughout the year to help screen students who might be at risk. It is also important to know what the expected level of performance is at the end of the year in order to determine how much growth we can expect a student to make compared to where she is starting. Benchmark scores are typically used for both of these purposes, helping to determine who is at risk and what is a reasonable end-of-year goal when setting up progress monitoring. While most curriculum-based measures provide benchmark scores that can be used for these purposes, there are still some measures that have not been benchmarked. Spelling is one of those measures that does not yet have benchmark scores associated with it. Therefore, the best way to determine expected level of performance three times a year as is done with universal screening and to determine end-of-year goals for progress monitoring is to use the 50% score on the norms for that grade for fall, winter, and spring. If a student scores below 50% on the norms, he would be considered being at risk in the area of spelling and could possibly benefit from additional instruction.

Norms for Spelling using CLS are presented in Table 5.1.

HOW DO I USE THE INFORMATION
TO WRITE SPELLING IEP GOALS AND OBJECTIVES?

Writing goals and objectives is a helpful way to define the behavior of interest and how it will be measured in order to be able to make decisions about a students learning. Chapter 2 provides the seven steps needed to write a good goal or objective. The seven steps include: time, learner, behavior, level, content, material, and criteria. Here, we will provide only an

TABLE 5.1. Norms for Spelling CBM: Correct Letter Sequences (CLS)

Grade	Percentile	aimsweb (2015)		
		Fall (CLS)	Winter (CLS)	Spring (CLS)
1	90%	46	53	56
	75%	41	49	53
	50%	**34**	**44**	**47**
	25%	24	38	41
	10%	11	31	35
2	90%	63	67	67
	75%	57	64	66
	50%	**49**	**56**	**62**
	25%	38	45	56
	10%	28	35	45
3	90%	105	109	111
	75%	98	104	108
	50%	**85**	**94**	**102**
	25%	67	78	90
	10%	46	59	70
4	90%	116	124	124
	75%	109	118	118
	50%	**95**	**110**	**111**
	25%	76	96	97
	10%	52	75	78
5	90%	137	137	138
	75%	133	133	134
	50%	**121**	**123**	**125**
	25%	96	109	112
	10%	73	88	94
6	90%	143	141	147
	75%	136	134	142
	50%	**126**	**123**	**132**
	25%	106	107	120
	10%	84	90	102
7	90%	134	143	146
	75%	124	136	141
	50%	**108**	**126**	**132**
	25%	90	110	118
	10%	72	92	101
8	90%	147	144	144
	75%	141	138	138
	50%	**134**	**128**	**128**
	25%	122	113	117
	10%	105	98	101

example for Spelling CBM but we encourage you to look at Chapter 2 for further information.

Example of Goals
- Spelling goal
  - In 30 weeks, Roberto will spell words from a fourth-grade spelling list from Spelling CBM progress monitoring material at 70 CLS in 2 minutes with greater than 95% accuracy.

The same principles apply to writing objectives, but one should use a shorter time frame.

Example of Objectives
- Spelling objective
  - In 10 weeks, Roberto will spell words from a fourth-grade spelling list from Spelling CBM progress monitoring material at 25 CLS in 2 minutes with greater than 95% accuracy.

FREQUENTLY ASKED QUESTIONS ABOUT SPELLING CBM

1. *Can I give students the list prior to the assessment?* No. This assessment is a general measure of students' skill at applying the spelling rules they have previously been taught. Giving students the list prior to the assessment increases the chance that they will attempt to memorize the words instead of learning the spelling skills being taught.

2. *The list for this week doesn't include the spelling rules I just taught. Can I choose one that does?* No. Avoid teaching to the test and remember Spelling CBM is designed to assess general, not specific, skill mastery.

3. *What if a student becomes distracted or fails to participate during the classroom administration?* Complete the classroom administration and then individually administer a different list at a later time.

4. *Not everyone in my class is on the same instructional level. Should I still give them all the same spelling list?* All students should be screened on their grade level, but they should be progress monitored on their instructional level, especially if they are receiving instruction on that level. The best way to handle this is to give both the grade-level and the instructional-level spelling lists each week so that you have an indication of how the students are doing given the instruction they are receiving (instructional level) and how well it is transferring to more difficult words (grade level).

5. *What if an interruption occurs during administration (e.g., fire alarm, school bell, class visitor)?* If a significant interruption occurs, stop administering the spelling list and administer a different list at a more appropriate time.

6. *Should I teach students the spelling rules they miss on the spelling lists?* Yes. Whenever students are missing previously taught rules, it is beneficial to reteach the material. This may be an indication that students did not fully understand the concept. Teachers should, however, continue to use the scope and sequence presented in the curriculum.

7. *What if I cannot tell what letter the student wrote?* In cases of doubt, do not give the student credit and be sure to tell her why. In extreme cases, administer another spelling list and ask the student to use her best handwriting.

8. *Can I use Spelling CBM for my students' weekly spelling test grade?* Yes. If your spelling curriculum matches the Spelling CBM lists (e.g., affixes, long vowels, compound words), it can be used for your weekly spelling test grade. You would want to make sure that the students and parents understand what the score means as well as what the goal for the year is.

9. *Can I use the norms to put students in instructional groups?* It is not recommended. Other assessment tools (e.g., Words Their Way spelling inventories) are more appropriate for identifying skill strengths and weaknesses in spelling. Instructional groupings will be more successful if they are based on student needs that can be used to guide instruction.

10. *If the student is not making progress, should I lower the goal?* No. Instead, assess the student's needs and provide additional interventions to address the target areas. How to do this is outlined in the troubleshooting chapter of *The ABCs of Curriculum-Based Evaluation* (Hosp, Hosp, Howell, & Allison, 2014).

11. *What should I do with the scored spelling sheets?* This information can be kept in a portfolio along with the graphed data to demonstrate progress over the year.

12. *I only have 20 Spelling CBM lists, but I need to progress monitor for 35 weeks. Is it OK to use the same lists again?* Yes. Once you have used all 20, start over using the first list again. The student probably doesn't remember specific words she spelled 20 weeks ago. This also means that you should not use the lists as homework or additional practice if you want to use them again.

RESOURCES AND/OR FURTHER READING

Fuchs, L. S., Allinder, R. M., & Hamlett, C. L. (1990). An analysis of spelling curricula and teachers' skills at identifying error types. *Remedial and Special Education, 11*(1), 42–52.

Fuchs, L. S., Fuchs, D., Hamlett, C. L., & Allinder, R. M. (1991). The contribution of skills analysis to curriculum-based measurement in spelling. *Exceptional Children, 57*, 443–452.

Robbins, K., Hosp, J., Hosp, M., & Flynn, L. (2010). Assessing specific grapho-phonemic skills in elementary students. *Assessment for Effective Intervention, 36*, 21–34.

Shinn, M. R., & Shinn, M. M. (2002). *AIMSweb training workbook: Administration and scoring of spelling curriculum-based measurement (S-CBM) for use in general outcome measurement.* Eden Prairie, MN: Edformation.

CHAPTER 6

How to Conduct Writing CBM

WHY SHOULD I CONDUCT WRITING CBM?

Writing is a critical skill that students need to master in order to succeed in school and life. Fortunately, there are specific skills that provide good indications of students' overall writing skills, allowing one to determine what writing skills they have mastered as well as to monitor their progress. As with all other CBM tasks, this information provides a database for each student so that appropriate instructional decisions can be made in a timely manner. We know that monitoring students' progress and making instructional decisions based on their progress leads to better outcomes for students. So what is Writing CBM?

Writing CBM has traditionally been made up of a short, simple measure of students' writing skill that requires students to write for 3 minutes on an instructional-level story starter. The response is then scored using multiple metrics, the most common being total words written (TWW), words spelled correctly (WSC), and correct writing sequences (CWS). There have been some advances in Writing CBM that we will mention here. However, since there are fewer studies available to support these new techniques, we will only cover the more common administration and scoring procedure below.

Some of the new advances include having students copy letters, words, and sentences; writing words beginning with a certain letter; picture word prompts; picture–theme prompts; and photo prompts (Lembke, Deno, & Hall, 2003; McMaster, Du, & Petursdottir, 2009; Ritchey, 2006). Each of these prompts requires the student to either write letters, words, sentences, or multiple sentences within 3 or 5 minutes' time. They are then scored using traditional CBM scoring procedure with the addition of some new scoring criteria like correct minus incorrect word sequences or total correct punctuation along with some qualitative indicators about the writing (Gansle, Noell, VanDerHeyden, Naquin, & Slider, 2002; Videen, Deno, & Marston, 1982). Writing CBM has been used successfully with secondary students (Espin, Scierka, Skare, & Halverson, 1999), middle school students (Espin et al., 2000), elementary students (Deno, Mirkin, Lowry, & Kuehnle, 1980; Deno, Marston, & Mirkin, 1982; Videen et al., 1982), and students with learning disabilities (Watkinson & Lee, 1992), as well as with students in kindergarten (Coker & Ritchey, 2010).

MATERIALS NEEDED TO CONDUCT WRITING CBM

1. Different but equivalent story starters that are grade appropriate.
2. Directions for administering and scoring Writing CBM.
3. Lined paper and writing utensils for student responses.
4. A stopwatch or countdown timer that displays seconds.
5. A quiet testing environment to work with students.
6. An equal-interval graph or a graphing program to plot the data.

WRITING CBM STORY STARTERS

The story starters should be equivalent in grade level and should be of the same interest for that grade. Story starters are short oral or written sentences that begin the writing process. They are designed to elicit more than a yes/no or short-answer response. The story starters should also elicit the writing skills the students are expected to master throughout the school year. While the story starters should be different, they should all be of equivalent difficulty (i.e., at the same grade level). The best way to assure this is to purchase generic story starters that have been developed specifically for this purpose. Sources for obtaining story starters are provided in Box 6.1. In addition, Figure 6.1 lists some story starters we have used.

BOX 6.1. Where to Find Premade Writing CBM Story Starters

$ indicates there is a cost for the story starters and/or graphing program.
⌨ indicates computerized administration available.
✎ indicates data management and graphing available.
S indicates Spanish measures are available.

aimsweb (Pearson) $⌨

Website: *www.aimsweb.com*
Phone: 866-313-6194
Products: Writing story starters

Intervention Central

Website: *www.interventioncentral.org*
Products: Writing story starters

Primary
- The funniest thing I did this summer was . . .
- The best part about school is . . .
- Today I woke up and . . .
- Yesterday I made a beautiful . . .
- The scariest Halloween I had was . . .
- The best vacation I ever took was . . .
- The dog was barking so loud that . . .
- Yesterday the class went to the zoo and . . .
- I was walking home from school one day when . . .
- I was walking to school one day when . . .
- My favorite game to play during recess is . . .
- If I could fly I would go . . .
- A little worm was crawling down the sidewalk when he . . .
- The dog climbed on the table and . . .
- There are many fun things to do at the park like . . .
- The best vacation I ever had was . . . .
- I could not find my puppy anywhere. I . . .
- I could not find my kitty anywhere. I . . .
- My dog saw a cat. I called out . . .
- At the circus I saw an elephant that was . . .
- When I was flying on a magic carpet . . .
- My favorite toy is . . .
- He knew something was different when . . .
- I looked out my window and to my surprise . . .
- On my way home from school I found a . . .

Intermediate
- I had never been afraid of being home alone at night until . . .
- "What is it?" I whispered to my friend, when suddenly . . .
- The lights went out and . . .
- I couldn't believe I had been voted class president! My first item of business was . . .
- When the alarm sounded I . . .
- I opened the front door and found a huge package and . . .
- One morning I woke up and sitting at the end of my bed was . . .
- As soon as I saw the large dog I knew . . .
- The dancer came onto the stage and . . .
- My day was going bad until . . .
- One day in the cafeteria, I saw some food on the ground . . .
- The dog looked sick and I heard sirens but saw no one . . .
- I looked out the window and to my surprise the world was white. Everything was covered with a blanket of snow. I . . .
- I saw the lighting and then I heard the thunder. I thought . . .
- Instead of going to bed last night, I decided to . . .

(continued)

FIGURE 6.1. Example of story starters for Writing CBM.

- While I was in my bed sleeping last night, I was awoken by . . .
- He knew something was different when . . .
- I was walking to school when . . .
- Out of a hole in the ground arose a great big . . .
- As I was walking through the cemetery I could hear . . .

Advanced
- It was like a dream come true when I . . .
- I knew I was in trouble when I couldn't find . . .
- "I knew it was you," I shouted when I noticed that . . .
- Once the noise stopped, everyone began to look around for what it was. It seemed to be . . .
- We arrived at the hotel expecting to be greeted, but instead . . .
- Number seven was winding up for the pitch when all of a sudden . . .
- Joe and Bob slowly crept up the creaky stairs and knocked on the door of the old house when . . .
- The teenagers were hiking through the forest when they came across an old rundown cabin that was . . .
- The light shined faintly through the fog, making it difficult to . . .
- The clerk at the store was annoyed, because . . .
- My dog was running toward the President and was about to . . .
- I could not sleep last night because . . .
- The funniest trick I ever played on _____ was . . .
- The waves were enormous and wind furious when all of a sudden . . .
- When I was swimming in the lake, I noticed . . .
- As I was coming out of the long tunnel, I happened to see . . .
- Mrs. Smith doesn't understand. I was only trying to . . .

FIGURE 6.1. *(continued)*

Just like the other curriculum-based measures, the first time Writing CBM is administered three equivalent story starters should be used, whether you are going to be conducting universal screening or progress monitoring. This should be conducted in one testing session, but it can occur across consecutive days if needed. We recommend doing it in one session to save setup time and obtain a more accurate score. The median score of these three samples will be used to provide the first data point on the student's graph. After that, 20–30 different but equivalent story starters will be used to monitor student progress in writing throughout the year.

Writing CBM can be administered individually or to a group. The story starters will be needed along with the directions and a timer. The student(s) should have lined paper and a pencil or pen. It may be helpful to give each student a spiral notebook for student responses. This allows teachers and students to see progress over time as well as provide a record of student responses. It is also helpful in situations where the measure is given to all students each week even though just a few are being progress monitored. See Figure 6.2 for an example of a student's response to the story starter "The best birthday I ever had was . . ."

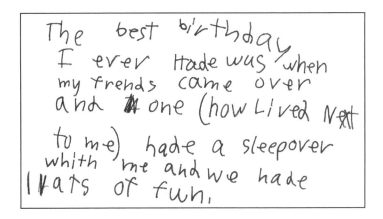

FIGURE 6.2. Example of student Writing CBM.

DIRECTIONS AND SCORING PROCEDURES FOR WRITING CBM

For your convenience, Appendix B includes a reproducible version of the directions and scoring rules for Writing CBM.

Directions for Writing CBM[1]

1. Provide students with a pencil and piece of lined paper or writing notebook.
2. Select an appropriate story starter.
3. Say: *"Today I want you to write a story. I am going to read a sentence to you first and then I want you to compose a short story about what happens. You will have 1 minute to think about what you will write and 3 minutes to write your story. Remember to do your best work. If you do not know how to spell a word, you should guess. Are there any questions?* (Pause) *Put your pencils down and listen. For the next minute, think about . . .* (insert story starter)."
4. After reading the story starter, begin your stopwatch and allow 1 minute for the student(s) to think. (*Monitor students so that they do not begin writing.*) After 30 seconds say: *"You should be thinking about . . .* (insert story starter)." At the end of 1 minute, restart your stopwatch for 3 minutes and say: *"Now begin writing."*
5. Monitor students' attention to the task. Encourage the students to work if they are not writing.
6. After 90 seconds say: *"You should be writing about . . .* (insert story starter)."
7. At the end of 3 minutes say: *"Thank you. Put your pencils down."*

Scoring Writing CBM

1. Count the total number of words written to obtain the TWW score.
2. Count the total number of words spelled correctly and subtract that from the TWW to obtain the WSC score.
3. Count the total number of correct writing sequences to obtain the CWS score.

---

[1]Adapted with permission from aimsweb (Powell-Smith & Shinn, 2004).

Each of the scores for TWW, WSC, and CWS provides a different way to evaluate a student's writing, and they should be looked at together. TWW is helpful from the broad perspective of the number of words written, while WSC and CWS help evaluate each word a student writes. Both TWW and WSC are scored without taking into consideration the context, or sophistication of what is produced. Only CWS provides for a more discrete scoring opportunity that takes into account meaning, punctuation, grammar, syntax, and semantics as well as spelling and punctuation.

Scoring Total Words Written (TWW)

- TWW is the number of words written regardless of spelling or context. When scoring TWW, the scorer <u>underlines</u> <u>each</u> <u>word</u> <u>written</u> and records the total number of words written (see Figure 6.3). Words are defined as any letter or group of letters, including misspelled or nonsense words, that have a space before and after them.
  - Student writes: I read the book.
  - Scored as: <u>I</u> <u>read</u> <u>the</u> <u>book</u>. = 4 total words written.
  - Student writes: I red the book.
  - Scored as: <u>I</u> <u>red</u> <u>the</u> <u>book</u>. = 4 total words written.
  - Student writes: I wont to go.
  - Scored as: <u>I</u> <u>wont</u> <u>to</u> <u>go</u>. = 4 total words written.
  - Student writes: I wanna go.
  - Scored as: <u>I</u> <u>wanna</u> <u>go</u>. = 3 total words written.
  - Student writes: Iv grqx zznip.
  - Scored as: <u>Iv</u> <u>grqx</u> <u>zznip</u>. = 3 total words written.

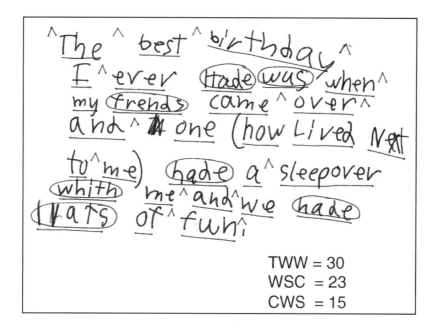

TWW = 30
WSC = 23
CWS = 15

FIGURE 6.3. Example of student Writing CBM scored.

- Abbreviations: Common abbreviations are counted as words (e.g., Dr., Mrs., TV).
  - Student writes: Dr. Smith came in.
  - Scored as: <u>Dr.</u> <u>Smith</u> <u>came</u> <u>in</u>. = 4 total words written.
  - Student writes: I like TV.
  - Scored as: <u>I</u> <u>like</u> <u>TV</u>. = 3 total words written.
- Hyphenated words: Each morpheme in a hyphenated word separated by a hyphen is counted as an individual word if it can stand alone. Prefixes separated by a hyphen are not counted as words, although the root word is counted.
  - Student writes: My sister-in-law came to visit.
  - Scored as: <u>My</u> <u>sister-in-law</u> <u>came</u> <u>to</u> <u>visit</u>. = 7 total words written.
  - Student writes: It is cold-blooded.
  - Scored as: <u>It</u> <u>is</u> <u>cold</u>-<u>blooded</u>. = 4 total words written.
  - Student writes: I love to bar-b-que.
  - Scored as: <u>I</u> <u>love</u> <u>to</u> <u>bar-b-que</u>. = 4 total words written.
  - Student writes: We need to re-evaluate the cost.
  - Scored as: <u>We</u> <u>need</u> <u>to</u> <u>re-evaluate</u> <u>the</u> <u>cost</u>. = 6 total words written.
- Titles and endings: Story titles and endings are counted as words written.
  - Student writes: My Bad Day by Sarah
  - Scored as: <u>My</u> <u>Bad</u> <u>Day</u> <u>by</u> <u>Sarah</u> = 5 total words written.
  - Student writes: The end.
  - Scored as: <u>The</u> <u>end</u>. = 2 total words written.
- Numerals: Numerals, with the exception of dates and currency, are not counted as words unless they are written out (i.e., as words).
  - Student writes: I have 3 cats.
  - Scored as: <u>I</u> <u>have</u> 3 <u>cats</u>. = 3 total words written.
  - Student writes: I have three cats.
  - Scored as: <u>I</u> <u>have</u> <u>three</u> <u>cats</u>. = 4 total words written.
  - Student writes: Today is August 13, 2016.
  - Scored as: <u>Today</u> <u>is</u> <u>August</u> <u>13</u>, <u>2016</u>. = 5 total words written.
  - Student writes: I have $50.
  - Scored as: <u>I</u> <u>have</u> <u>$50</u>. = 3 total words written.
  - Student writes: I have 50.
  - Scored as: <u>I</u> <u>have</u> 50. = 2 total words written.
  - Student writes: I have 50 dollars.
  - Scored as: <u>I</u> <u>have</u> <u>50</u> <u>dollars</u>. = 4 total words written.
- Unusual characters: Unusual characters are not counted as words even if they are meant to take the place of a word.
  - Student writes: Mary & I went home.
  - Scored as: <u>Mary</u> & <u>I</u> <u>went</u> <u>home</u>. = 4 total words written.
  - Student writes: She won a lot of $.
  - Scored as: <u>She</u> <u>won</u> <u>a</u> <u>lot</u> <u>of</u> $. = 5 total words written.
  - Student writes: I will give you 50%.
  - Scored as: <u>I</u> <u>will</u> <u>give</u> <u>you</u> 50%. = 4 total words written.

Scoring Words Spelled Correctly (WSC)

WSC is the number of correctly spelled words, regardless of context. Words are counted in WSC if they can be found in the English language. Incorrectly spelled words should be circled (see Figure 6.3). WSC is calculated by subtracting the total number of circled words from the TWW. As with TWW, additional scoring rules apply to WSC.

- Abbreviations: Abbreviations must be spelled correctly.
  - Student writes: I live on President Blvd.
  - Scored as: I live on President Blvd. = 5 words spelled correctly.
  - Student writes: I live on President Bld.
  - Scored as: I live on President (Bld.) = 4 words spelled correctly.
- Hyphenated words: Each morpheme counted as an individual word must be spelled correctly. If the morpheme cannot stand alone (e.g., prefix) and part of the word is incorrect, the entire word is counted as an incorrect spelling.
  - Student writes: She is my sister-in-law.
  - Scored as: She is my sister-in-law. = 6 words spelled correctly.
  - Student writes: She is my sista-in-law.
  - Scored as: She is my (sista)-in-law. = 5 words spelled correctly.
  - Student writes: I need to re-evaluate this.
  - Scored as: I need to re-evaluate this. = 5 words spelled correctly.
  - Student writes: I need to re-eveluate this.
  - Scored as: I need to (re-eveluate) this. = 4 words spelled correctly.
- Titles and endings: Words in the title or ending are counted in the words spelled correctly.
  - Student writes: My Terrible Day.
  - Scored as: My Terrible Day. = 3 words spelled correctly.
  - Student writes: My Terrable Day.
  - Scored as: My (Terrable) Day. = 2 words spelled correctly.
- Capitalization: Proper nouns must be capitalized unless the name is also a common noun. Capitalization of the first word in the sentence is not a requirement for the word to be spelled correctly. Words are counted as spelled correctly even if they are capitalized incorrectly within the sentence.
  - Student writes: She sat with Bill.
  - Scored as: She sat with Bill. = 4 words spelled correctly.
  - Student writes: she sat with Bill.
  - Scored as: she sat with Bill. = 4 words spelled correctly.
  - Student writes: She sat with bill.
  - Scored as: She sat with bill. = 4 words spelled correctly.
  - Student writes: She sat with the bill.
  - Scored as: She sat with the bill. = 5 words spelled correctly.
  - Student writes: She sat With the bill.
  - Scored as: She sat With the bill. = 5 words spelled correctly.

- Reversed letters: Words containing letter reversals are not counted as errors unless the reversal causes the word to be spelled incorrectly. This typically applies with reversals of the following letters: *p, q, g, d, b, n, u*.
    - Student writes: The pig was at the farm.
    - Scored as: The pig was at the farm. = 6 words spelled correctly.
    - Student writes: The qig was at the farm.
    - Scored as: The (qig) was at the farm. = 5 words spelled correctly.
    - Student writes: The big pig ate.
    - Scored as: The big pig ate. = 4 words spelled correctly.
    - Student writes: The dig pig ate.
    - Scored as: The dig pig ate. = 4 words spelled correctly.
- Contractions: In order for a contraction to be counted as correct, it must have the apostrophe in the correct place unless the word can stand alone.
    - Student writes: Its my turn.
    - Scored as: Its my turn. = 3 words spelled correctly.
    - Student writes: It's my turn.
    - Scored as: It's my turn. = 3 words spelled correctly.
    - Student writes: She isn't here.
    - Scored as: She isn't here. = 3 words spelled correctly.
    - Student writes: She isnt here.
    - Scored as: She (isnt) here. = 2 words spelled correctly.

Scoring Correct Writing Sequences (CWS)

A CWS is "two adjacent, correctly spelled words that are acceptable within the context of the [written] phrase to a native speaker of the English language" (Videen et al., 1982, p. 7). It takes into account punctuation, syntax, semantics, spelling, and capitalization. When scoring CWS, a caret (^) is used to mark each correct word sequence. A space is implied at the beginning of a sentence. The following should be taken into consideration when scoring CWS.

- Spelling: Words must be spelled correctly to be counted in CWS. Words that are not counted in WSC or are circled words are *not* counted as correct writing sequences.
    - Student writes: She waited for me at the store.
    - Scored as: ^She^waited^for^me^at^the^store^. = 8 correct writing sequences.
    - Student writes: She waeted for me at the stor.
    - Scored as: ^She waeted for^me^at^the stor. = 4 correct writing sequences.
- Capitalization: Capitalization at the beginning of the sentence is necessary. Proper nouns must be capitalized unless they can serve as common nouns in the given context. Incorrectly capitalized words are marked as incorrect CWS.
    - Student writes: She is coming over.
    - Scored as: ^She^is^coming^over^. = 5 correct writing sequences.
    - Student writes: she is coming over.
    - Scored as: she is^coming^over^. = 3 correct writing sequences.

- Student writes: She sat with bill.
- Scored as: ^She^sat^with bill. = 3 correct writing sequences.
- Student writes: She sat with the bill.
- Scored as: ^She^sat^with^the^bill^. = 6 correct writing sequences.
- Student writes: He is on my Pillow.
- Scored as: ^He^is^on^my Pillow. = 4 correct writing sequences.

- Punctuation: Punctuation at the end of the sentence must be correct. Commas are not typically counted unless they are used in a series. In a series, they must be used correctly to be scored. Other punctuation marks are typically not counted as CWS.
  - Student writes: Mary asked if I would come over. I said no.
  - Scored as: ^Mary^asked^if^I^would^come^over^.^I^said^no^. = 12 correct writing sequences.
  - Student writes: Mary asked if I would come over i said no.
  - Scored as: ^Mary^asked^if^I^would^come ^over i^said^no. = 9 correct writing sequences.
  - Student writes: I have a cat, dog and bird.
  - Scored as: ^I^have^a^cat,^dog^and^bird^. = 8 correct writing sequences.
  - Student writes: I have a cat dog and bird.
  - Scored as: ^I^have^a^cat dog^and^bird^. = 7 correct writing sequences.

- Syntax: Words must be syntactically correct to be counted as CWS. Sentences that begin with a conjunction are considered to be syntactically correct.
  - Student writes: He had never seen the movie before.
  - Scored as: ^He^had^never^seen^the^movie^before^. = 8 correct writing sequences.
  - Student writes: He never seen the movie ever.
  - Scored as: ^He^never seen^the^movie ever^. = 5 correct writing sequences.
  - Student writes: And he wanted to go see it with me.
  - Scored as: ^And^he^wanted^to^go^see^it^with^me^. = 10 correct writing sequences.

- Semantics: Words must be semantically correct to be counted in CWS.
  - Student writes: That pig is too fat.
  - Scored as: ^That^pig^is^too^fat^. = 6 correct writing sequences.
  - Student writes: That pig is to fat.
  - Scored as: ^That^pig^is to fat^. = 4 correct writing sequences.

- Story titles and endings: Story titles and endings are included in the scoring of CWS and must meet scoring criteria for spelling, punctuation, capitalization, syntax, and semantics to be counted in CWS.
  - Student writes: The Big Fat Wedding by Billy
  - Scored as: ^The^Big^Fat^Wedding^by^Billy^ = 7 correct writing sequences.
  - Student writes: The Big fat Wedding by billy
  - Scored as: ^The^Big fat Wedding^by billy = 3 correct writing sequences.
  - Student writes: the big fat wedding
  - Scored as: the big fat wedding = 0 correct writing sequences.
  - Student writes: The End.
  - Scored as: ^The^End^. = 3 correct writing sequences.

- Student writes: The end.
- Scored as: ^The end^. = 2 correct writing sequences.

Special Administration and Scoring Considerations for Writing CBM

1. Correction procedure: If the student makes an error, he is *not* corrected.
2. Discontinuation rule: There is no discontinuation rule for Writing CBM.
3. Although TWW and WSC are easy to score, they tend to yield fluency information only. The extra time needed to score CWS is suggested at all levels for students below grade level in writing. CWS scoring supplies a great deal of useful information about error patterns and missing skills. It is also more sensitive to instruction, so it makes a better tool for progress monitoring.
4. Directions should be read as presented above, and students should not receive additional instructions or corrections during any part of the test administration.
5. Test administrators may find that 3-minute written responses do not yield enough information, particularly for students struggling with writing. Longer samples using 5 and 10 minutes can be used for analysis, but the scores cannot be used in comparison to the norm if the normative sample used 3 minutes. Another option is to note where the student is at the end of 3 minutes to compare to the normative sample but then let him keep writing for an additional 2–7 minutes.

HOW OFTEN SHOULD WRITING CBM BE ADMINISTERED?

In Chapter 2, we provide additional details on how often and when to administer CBM for the different purposes of universal screening and progress monitoring. Below we provide an outline for universal screening and progress monitoring for Writing CBM. We suggest you refer to Chapter 2 for a more in-depth discussion on how often and when to give CBM for these different purposes.

Universal Screening

All students should be screened using grade level materials three times a year. This typically occurs in Fall, Winter, and Spring. Universal screening data assist in answering some important questions, two of which are:

"Is this student *at risk* for academic failure by the end of the year?"
"Is our core instruction meeting the needs of most of our students?"

Progress Monitoring

Only those students who have been identified as *at risk*, meaning they did not score at or above the benchmark score on the universal screening assessment, should be progress monitored at least once a week on instructional level material and at least once per month on grade level materials if it is different from instructional level. An important aspect of progress monitoring is to do it often (i.e., weekly) and consistently (i.e., using CBM materials that are at the same difficulty level). Progress monitoring data assist in answering two very important questions:

"Is this student benefiting from the instruction he is receiving?"
"Is this intervention helping the majority of the students who have received it?"

HOW MUCH TIME DOES IT TAKE TO ADMINISTER AND SCORE WRITING CBM?

It takes approximately 5 minutes to administer a writing sample to an individual or a whole group. The time needed for scoring Writing CBM depends on the number of measures scored and the grade level of the students (the time needed increases with grade level). Malecki and Jewell (2003) found that it took an average of 30 seconds to score a single fluency measure (TWW or WSC). When two fluency measures (TWW and CWS) were scored, the time increased to a little less than a minute for elementary grades and just over a minute for middle school grades. The time increased to 1½ minutes for early elementary student levels and 2½ minutes for middle school student levels when all three measures (TWW, WSC, and CWS) were scored. If only CWS is scored, an average of 45 seconds to 1½ minutes is needed.

WRITING CBM SCORES

It is important to know what the expected level of performance is throughout the year to help screen students who might be at risk. It is also important to know what the expected level of performance is at the end of the year in order to determine how much growth we can expect a student to make compared to where she is starting. Benchmark scores are typically used for both of these purposes, helping to determine who is at risk and what is a reasonable end of year goal when setting up progress monitoring. While most curriculum-based measures provide benchmark scores that can be used for these purposes there are still some measures that have not been benchmarked. Like spelling, writing is another one of those curriculum-based measures that does not yet have benchmark scores associated with it. Therefore, the best way to determine expected level of performance three times a year as is done with universal screening and to determine end-of-year goals for progress monitoring is to use the 50% score on the norms for that grade for fall, winter, and spring. If a student scores below 50% on the norms, he would be considered being at risk in the area of writing and could possibly benefit from additional instruction.

Norms for Writing using CWS, TWW, and WSC are presented in Tables 6.1–6.3.

TABLE 6.1. Norms for Writing CBM: Correct Writing Sequences (CWS)

Grade	Percentile	aimsweb (2015)		
		Fall (CWS)	Winter (CWS)	Spring (CWS)
K	90%	12	16	19
	75%	8	12	15
	50%	**4**	**7**	**9**
	25%	1	1	3
	10%	0	0	1
1	90%	7	16	26
	75%	4	10	18
	50%	**2**	**5**	**11**
	25%	1	2	5
	10%	0	1	2
2	90%	23	36	39
	75%	15	25	30
	50%	**9**	**16**	**21**
	25%	4	9	13
	10%	2	5	8
3	90%	38	48	56
	75%	27	35	43
	50%	**18**	**24**	**30**
	25%	11	15	21
	10%	5	9	13
4	90%	50	57	62
	75%	39	45	51
	50%	**28**	**34**	**38**
	25%	18	23	27
	10%	10	14	18
5	90%	56	63	69
	75%	44	52	57
	50%	**34**	**39**	**46**
	25%	24	28	32
	10%	15	19	22
6	90%	65	72	78
	75%	51	59	66
	50%	**37**	**47**	**53**
	25%	25	35	40
	10%	16	24	29
7	90%	71	73	76
	75%	60	62	66
	50%	**47**	**52**	**53**
	25%	35	40	42
	10%	23	29	31
8	90%	73	79	81
	75%	62	69	69
	50%	**49**	**56**	**56**
	25%	37	44	44
	10%	24	31	35

TABLE 6.2. Norms for Writing CBM: Words Spelled Correct (WSC)

Grade	Percentile	aimsweb (2015)		
		Fall (WSC)	Winter (WSC)	Spring (WSC)
K	90%	17	11	16
	75%	3	5	10
	50%	**1**	**2**	**6**
	25%	0	1	3
	10%	0	0	1
1	90%	14	22	31
	75%	9	15	23
	50%	**5**	**10**	**16**
	25%	2	5	10
	10%	1	2	5
2	90%	23	39	42
	75%	16	29	33
	50%	**10**	**21**	**24**
	25%	6	12	17
	10%	3	6	11
3	90%	38	47	54
	75%	30	38	43
	50%	**21**	**28**	**33**
	25%	13	18	23
	10%	8	11	16
4	90%	51	55	57
	75%	41	45	46
	50%	**30**	**35**	**35**
	25%	21	25	25
	10%	13	17	17
5	90%	57	63	75
	75%	48	51	62
	50%	**36**	**40**	**49**
	25%	26	29	38
	10%	18	20	27
6	90%	68	76	76
	75%	57	63	66
	50%	**44**	**50**	**56**
	25%	32	40	45
	10%	20	30	35
7	90%	82	72	82
	75%	70	63	73
	50%	**52**	**52**	**63**
	25%	39	40	51
	10%	27	30	41
8	90%	77	83	93
	75%	69	72	82
	50%	**55**	**60**	**71**
	25%	43	48	60
	10%	26	36	48

TABLE 6.3. Norms for Writing CBM: Total Words Written (TWW)

Grade	Percentile	aimsweb (2015)		
		Fall (TWW)	Winter (TWW)	Spring (TWW)
K	90%	10	16	20
	75%	3	10	14
	50%	**1**	**5**	**10**
	25%	1	2	6
	10%	0	1	3
1	90%	17	26	35
	75%	12	19	28
	50%	**7**	**13**	**20**
	25%	4	8	14
	10%	2	5	9
2	90%	30	42	49
	75%	22	34	41
	50%	**15**	**25**	**32**
	25%	10	18	24
	10%	5	11	16
3	90%	44	53	59
	75%	35	44	49
	50%	**26**	**34**	**39**
	25%	19	25	30
	10%	13	17	23
4	90%	55	60	66
	75%	45	51	56
	50%	**35**	**41**	**45**
	25%	26	31	35
	10%	17	22	25
5	90%	60	68	74
	75%	51	59	63
	50%	**41**	**48**	**51**
	25%	30	37	41
	10%	21	27	31
6	90%	71	78	85
	75%	58	66	73
	50%	**46**	**55**	**59**
	25%	35	43	47
	10%	24	33	36
7	90%	79	84	87
	75%	67	72	74
	50%	**53**	**60**	**61**
	25%	42	48	48
	10%	32	37	37
8	90%	90	81	90
	75%	78	70	79
	50%	**63**	**59**	**69**
	25%	50	49	58
	10%	38	38	47

HOW DO I USE THE INFORMATION
TO WRITE WRITING IEP GOALS AND OBJECTIVES?

Writing goals and objectives are a helpful way to define the behavior of interest and how it will be measured in order to be able to make decisions about a students learning. Chapter 2 provides the seven steps needed to write a good goal or objective. The seven steps include: time, learner, behavior, level, content, material, and criteria. Here, we will provide only an example for Writing CBM but we encourage you to look at Chapter 2 for further information.

Example of Goals

- Writing goal
  - In 30 weeks, Jose will write from sixth-grade writing story starter CBM progress monitoring material at 47 CWS in 3 minutes with greater than 95% accuracy.

The same principles apply to writing objectives, but one should use a shorter time frame.

Example of Objectives

- Writing objective
  - In 10 weeks, Jose will write from sixth-grade writing story starter CBM progress monitoring material at 30 CWS in 3 minutes with greater than 95% accuracy.

FREQUENTLY ASKED QUESTIONS ABOUT WRITING CBM

1. *What do you do if a student stops writing before the time is up?* You should say to the student: **"Keep writing the best story you can."** This prompt can be used as many times as needed.

2. *Does it matter that a student's response does not relate to the story starter?* No. Responses are not scored for content, organization, or detail. You would, however, want to note this and make sure that the student understands the story starters or has the background knowledge to be able to write on the topic.

3. *Can I change the directions or how I score the student responses?* No. The directions are already short and provide you with a standard procedure to follow. Even though they may not seem to be using it productively, it is especially important to give the students 1 minute of think time before they begin to write.

4. *Can I create my own story starters?* Yes, as long as they are appropriate for the grade level and elicit more than a yes/no response. This can also offer an opportunity to incorporate students' interests in the writing task.

5. *What if a student does not start writing even though I know he is capable of doing so?* Encourage the student to begin writing. Let the student know what the expectations are. If necessary, implement instructional or behavioral techniques to address the student's area of need.

6. *What if I cannot read the student's writing?* Assess if the student needs instruction in handwriting or if it is just carelessness. Then provide interventions to address the problem (e.g., handwriting practice, motivational tools). Administer additional story starters as necessary.

7. *Can students score each other's responses?* No. Students can score their own TWW, but the other measures should be scored by the teacher or someone trained in Writing CBM.

8. *Can I use student responses on Writing CBM to give grades?* This can be done if you also include an additional scoring procedure (e.g., a rubric) that looks at the content you are teaching.

9. *Can I use the norms to put students in instructional groups?* It is not recommended unless additional information is collected that aligns with what you are teaching and identifies skill strengths and weaknesses in writing. Instructional groupings will be more successful if they are based on student needs that can be used to guide instruction.

10. *If the student is not making progress, should I lower the goal?* No. Instead, assess the student's needs and provide additional interventions to address the target areas. How to do this is outlined in the troubleshooting chapter of *The ABCs of Curriculum-Based Evaluation* (Hosp et al., 2014).

11. *What should I do with the scored stories?* This information can be kept in a portfolio along with the graphed data to demonstrate progress over the year. Students can also use their responses as starting points for longer writing assignments.

12. *I only have 20 CBM story starters, but I need to progress monitor for 35 weeks. Is it OK to use the same story starters again?* Yes. Once you have used all 20, start using them again. The student probably doesn't remember specific items he did 20 weeks ago. This also means that you should not use the story starters for homework or additional practice if you want to use them again.

RESOURCES AND/OR FURTHER READING

Espin, C. A., Scierka, B. J., Skare, S., & Halverson, N. (1999). Criterion-related validity of curriculum-based measures in writing for secondary school students. *Reading and Writing Quarterly: Overcoming Learning Difficulties, 15*(1), 5–27.

Gansle, K. A., Noell, G. H., VanDerHeyden, A. M., Naquin, G. M., & Slider, N. J. (2002). Moving beyond total words written: The reliability, criterion validity, and time cost of alternate measures for curriculum-based measurement in writing. *School Psychology Review, 31*, 477–497.

Lembke, E., Deno, S. L., & Hall, K. (2003). Identifying an indicator of growth in early writing proficiency for elementary school students. *Assessment for Effective Intervention, 28*(3/4), 23–35.

Malecki, C. K., & Jewell, J. (2003). Developmental, gender, and practical considerations in scoring curriculum-based measurement writing probes. *Psychology in the Schools, 40*, 379–390.

Ritchey, K. D., & Coker, D. L. (2013). An investigation of the validity and utility of two curriculum-based measurement writing tasks. *Reading and Writing Quarterly, 29*, 89–119.

CHAPTER 7

How to Conduct
Early Numeracy CBM

WHY SHOULD I CONDUCT EARLY NUMERACY CBM?

Just as early literacy skills have gained prominence for assessment of reading (in order to prevent future problems), early numeracy skills are gaining prominence in math even though numeracy and math still have not reached the same level of awareness that early literacy and reading have. While Math CBM focuses on two components of math (computation using M-COMP and problem solving using M-CAP), Early Numeracy CBM focuses on the third component of math: number sense. Just as Early Reading CBM focuses on the foundational skills that must be mastered to automaticity to facilitate proficient reading, Early Numeracy CBM includes the foundational skills that must be mastered to automaticity to facilitate computation and problem solving in math.

Research on Early Numeracy CBM is still in its infancy, but there are several promising measures. One difficulty in the development of early numeracy curriculum-based measures is that there has not been enough work on conceptual understanding of early numeracy to fully specify which skills might serve as the best predictors of overall competence (Methe et al., 2011). However, there are a few measures that are showing promise: Counting CBM, Number Identification CBM, Missing Number CBM, Quantity Discrimination CBM, and Math Facts. The first four listed are described below, Math Facts is similar to the procedures discussed and provided in Chapter 8 for Math. To help you easily find Early Numeracy CBM materials we provide sources in Box 7.1.

COUNTING CBM

Counting is an important component of number sense not only because it measures automatic recall of number names, but because unlike letters, numbers are in a meaningful order. There are two general approaches to counting as an Early Numeracy CBM: Oral Counting CBM and Touch Counting CBM. Oral Counting CBM can be as simple as the

BOX 7.1. Where to Find Premade Early Numeracy CBM Sheets

$ indicates there is a cost for the materials and/or graphing program.
⌨ indicates computerized administration available.
✍ indicates data management and graphing available.

aimsweb (Pearson) $✍

Website: *www.aimsweb.com*

Phone: 866-313-6194

Products: • Oral Counting
          • Missing Number
          • Number Identification
          • Quantity Discrimination

FastBridge Learning $⌨✍

Website: *www.fastbridge.org*

Phone: 612-424-3714

Products: • Counting Objects
          • Number Identification

Intervention Central

Website: *www.interventioncentral.org*

Products: • Number Identification
          • Missing Number
          • Quantity Discrimination

mCLASS: Math $⌨✍

Website: *www.amplify.com*

Phone: 800-823-1969

Products: • Oral Counting
          • Missing Number
          • Number Identification
          • Quantity Discrimination

Research Institute on Progress Monitoring (RIPM)

Website: *www.progressmonitoring.org*

Phone: 612-626-7220

Products: • Number Identification
          • Missing Number
          • Quantity Discrimination

student counting orally starting at 1 and going as high as he can. Touch Counting CBM adds the dimension of one-to-one correspondence by including the action of associating each number with an item being counted.

Materials Needed to Conduct Counting CBM

1. A student prompt with up to 100 dots (Touch Counting CBM only; student and/or teacher/examiner copies).
2. Directions for administering and scoring Counting CBM.
3. A writing utensil and clipboard or computer to enter student responses.
4. A stopwatch or countdown timer that displays seconds.
5. A quiet testing environment to work with students.
6. An equal-interval graph or a graphing program to plot the data.

Counting CBM Sheets

Oral Counting CBM does not require any student specific prompts. Within the directions, the student is instructed to count. Most versions ask students to start at 1 and count as high as they can. Other approaches might include counting by 2s, 5s, or 10s. Touch Counting CBM sheets should include at least 100 identical items such as circles or dots. A printed prompt rather than manipulatives are recommended because consistency of order and all items being identical can be controlled. For the purposes of discussing the directions, scoring, and additional considerations, we will be referring to the aimsweb materials for Oral Counting CBM. We recommend readers look at the specific measures they will be using to ensure they follow the administration and scoring rules applicable for that specific measure, as there are variations among publishers.

We recommend administering all universal screening assessments in one testing session to save setup time and for consistency in obtaining an accurate score, but it can occur across consecutive days if needed. If three samples of the same CBM task are to be administered, then the median score is used for the final score and can also be placed as the first data point on the student's graph. After that, 20–30 different but equivalent sheets will be used to monitor student progress in reading throughout the year. Unlike many other CBMs, the first time Counting CBM is administered to the student(s), three equivalent sheets are not needed. No student materials are required for Oral Counting CBM, and only a single sheet is needed for Touch Counting CBM. In addition, the same Touch Counting CBM sheet can be used every time for progress monitoring (it's just a page of circles rather than different text or content).

Counting CBM must be administered individually. For Oral Counting CBM, no student sheet is needed (because it is all oral), but for Touch Counting CBM two copies of the sheet will be needed. The student should have a copy of the Touch Counting CBM sheet in front of her, and the teacher/examiner should either have a copy of the Counting CBM sheet in front of her on the computer screen or a paper copy to write on and a writing utensil, as well as a timer and the directions. See Figures 7.1, 7.2, and 7.3 for examples of each type of sheet.

Grade 1 AIMSweb Oral Counting									
1	2	3	4	5	6	7	8	9	10
11	12	13	14	15	16	17	18	19	20
21	22	23	24	25	26	27	28	29	30
31	32	33	34	35	36	37	38	39	40
41	42	43	44	45	46	47	48	49	50
51	52	53	54	55	56	57	58	59	60
61	62	63	64	65	66	67	68	69	70
71	72	73	74	75	76	77	78	79	80
81	82	83	84	85	86	87	88	89	90
91	92	93	94	95	96	97	98	99	100

Total Corrects: _____

FIGURE 7.1. Example of teacher/examiner Oral Counting CBM sheet. Reprinted with permission from aimsweb.

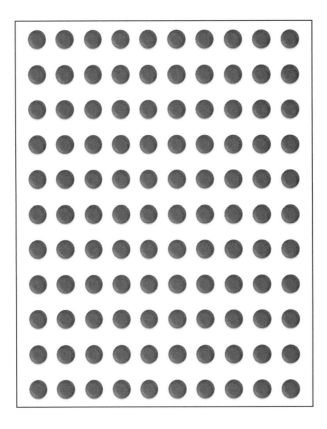

FIGURE 7.2. Example of student Touch Counting CBM sheet.

Student name:						Grade:	Date:		
1	2	3	4	5	6	7	8	9	10
11	12	13	14	15	16	17	18	19	20
21	22	23	24	25	26	27	28	29	30
31	32	33	34	35	36	37	38	39	40
41	42	43	44	45	46	47	48	49	50
51	52	53	54	55	56	57	58	59	60
61	62	63	64	65	66	67	68	69	70
71	72	73	74	75	76	77	78	79	80
81	82	83	84	85	86	87	88	89	90
91	92	93	94	95	96	97	98	99	100

FIGURE 7.3. Example of teacher/examiner Touch Counting CBM sheet.

Directions and Scoring Procedures for Counting CBM

For your convenience, Appendix B includes a reproducible version of the directions and scoring rules for both Oral Counting CBM and Touch Counting CBM.

Directions for Oral Counting CBM[1]

1. Place the teacher/examiner copy on the clipboard so the student cannot see it.
2. Say: ***"When I say 'Start' I want you to start counting aloud from 1, like this: 1, 2, 3, until I tell you to stop. If you come to a number you don't know, I'll tell it to you. Be sure to do your best counting. Ready? Start."*** (*Trigger timer for 1 minute.*)
3. Follow along on the teacher/examiner copy as the student counts and put a slash (/) through any incorrect or skipped numbers.
4. At the end of 1 minute say ***"Stop"*** and put a bracket (]) after the last number counted.

Directions for Touch Counting CBM

1. Place a copy of the student sheet in front of the student.
2. Place the teacher/examiner copy on the clipboard so the student cannot see it.

---

[1]Adapted with permission from aimsweb (Shinn & Shinn, 2002a).

3. Say: *"When I say 'Begin' I want you to start counting from the top of the page* (point to the first dot) *until I tell you to stop. Count across the page. When you come to the end of a row, go to the next row. If you come to a number you don't know, I'll tell it to you. Be sure to do your best counting. Ready? Begin."* (Trigger timer for 1 minute.)

4. Follow along on the teacher/examiner copy as the student counts and put a slash (/) through any incorrect or skipped numbers.

5. At the end of 1 minute say: *"Please stop"* and put a bracket (]) after the last number counted.

Scoring Oral and Touch Counting CBM

Submit the results using the online system. Or:

1. Count the total number of numbers attempted.
2. Count the total number of errors.
3. Calculate rate: Total items attempted – total errors = total correct per minute.
4. Calculate accuracy: Total correct ÷ total items attempted = percent correct.

SCORED AS CORRECT

Oral Counting CBM and Touch Counting CBM are scored based on each number that is stated correctly or touched correctly as it is associated with a correct number amount. Each correct response counts toward the total score defined as the total number correct (NC).

- Pronounced/answered correctly: A number must be correctly pronounced in the correct order. For Touch Counting CBM, it also must be associated with the pointing to or touching of one circle.
  - *Example:* 2, 3, 4, 5
    - Student says: 2, 3, 4, 6
    - Scored as: 3 NC (2, 3, 4, 6̸)
- Self-corrections within 3 seconds: Numbers miscounted initially but corrected within 3 seconds are scored as correct. If already slashed as an error, the number is circled.
  - *Example:* 5, 6, 7, 8, 9
    - Student says: 5, 6, 8, 9 . . . 7, 8, 9
    - Scored as: 5 NC (5, 6, ⑦ 8, 9)
- Dialect/articulation: Variations in pronunciation explainable by local language norms or speech sound production.
  - *Example:* 7
    - Student says: /seb-en/ instead of /sev-en/; this would be accepted if this is due to an articulation problem.
    - Scored as: 1 NC
- Repetitions: Repeating the same number(s) more than once before moving on.
  - *Example:* 5, 6, 7, 8, 9
    - Student says: 5, 6, 7 . . . 7, 8, 9
    - Scored as: 5 NC (5, 6, 7, 8, 9)

- Insertions: Adding a number that does not belong in the sequence.
  - *Example:* 5, 6, 7, 8, 9
    - Student says: 5, 6, 7, 26, 8, 9
    - Scored as: 5 NC (5, 6, 7, 8, 9)

SCORED AS ERRORS

All errors are marked with a slash (/) through the number.

- Mispronunciations/substitutions: When a nonnumber name or name of wrong number is given.
  - *Example: 11*
    - Student says: /oneteen/ instead of /eleven/.
    - Scored as: 0 NC (11̸)
- Omissions: Numbers that are not produced.
  - *Example:* 5, 6, 7, 8, 9
    - Student says: 5, 6, 8, 9
    - Scored as: 4 NC (5, 6, 7̸, 8, 9)
- Hesitations without response: Not responding for 3 seconds and being prompted by providing the number.
  - *Example:* 5, 6, 7, 8
    - Student says: 5, 6, 7 . . . (3 sec). Say: "**8**."
    - Scored as: 3 NC (5, 6, 7, 8̸)
- Hesitations with response: Starting to respond but not finishing within 3 seconds and being prompted by providing the number.
  - *Example:* 5, 6, 7
    - Student says: 5, 6, ssssssss (3 sec). Say: "**7**."
    - Scored as: 2 NC (5, 6, 7̸)
- Reversals: Transposing two or more numbers.
  - *Example:* 5, 6, 7, 8, 9
    - Student says: 5, 6, 8, 7, 9
    - Scored as: 3 NC (5, 6, 7̸, 8̸, 9)
- Skipped items: A number is skipped in a sequence and not stated.
  - *Example: 8, 9, 10, 11, 12, 13, 14, 15, 16, 17*
    - Student says: 8, 9, 10, 12, 15, 16, 17
    - Scored as: 7 NC (8, 9, 10, 11̸, 12, 13̸, 14̸, 15, 16, 17)

Special Administration and Scoring Considerations for Counting CBM

1. Correction procedure: If the student makes an error, she is not corrected. The only time a number is provided is if the student hesitates for 3 seconds.
2. Skip an entire row/line: If the student skips a row of numbers, the row is crossed out and each number is counted as an error.
3. Discontinuation rule: There is no discontinuation rule for Counting CBM.

NUMBER IDENTIFICATION CBM

Number Identification CBM is designed to assess number sense, which is a fundamental component of math skills. Similar to letter naming for Early Reading, number identification is a risk indicator for math because it measures automaticity.

Materials Needed to Conduct Number Identification CBM

1. Different but equivalent stimulus sheets (student and teacher/examiner copies).
2. Directions for administering and scoring Number ID.
3. A writing utensil and clipboard or computer to enter student responses.
4. A stopwatch or countdown timer that displays seconds.
5. A quiet testing environment to work with students.
6. An equal-interval graph or a graphing program to plot the data.

Number Identification CBM Sheets

Number Identification CBM sheets should have different items. For the purposes of discussing the directions, scoring, and additional considerations, we will be referring to the Research Institute on Progress Monitoring (RIPM) materials. We recommend you look at the specific measures you will be using to ensure you follow the administration and scoring rules applicable for that specific measure, as there are variations among publishers.

We recommend administering all universal screening assessments in one testing session to save setup time and for consistency in obtaining an accurate score, but it can occur across consecutive days if needed. If three samples of the same CBM task are to be administered, then the median score is used for the final score and can also be placed as the first data point on the student's graph. After that, 20–30 different but equivalent sheets will be used to monitor student progress in reading throughout the year.

Number Identification CBM must be administered individually. Two copies of the sheet will be needed. The student should have a copy of the Number Identification CBM sheet in front of him, and the teacher/examiner should either have a copy of the Number Identification CBM sheet in front of her on the computer screen or a paper copy to write on and a writing utensil, as well as a timer and the directions. See Figures 7.4 and 7.5 for examples of each type of sheet.

Directions and Scoring Procedures for Number Identification CBM

For your convenience, Appendix B includes a reproducible version of the directions and scoring rules for Number Identification CBM.

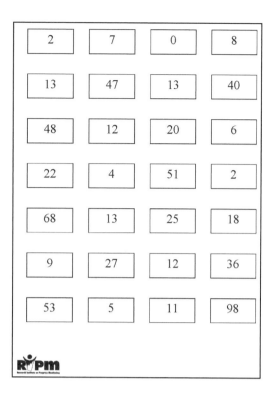

FIGURE 7.4. Example of student Number Identification CBM sheet. Reprinted with permission from Research Institute on Progress Monitoring.

Date: _____   Number Correct _____

Direction: Write the number that the student says in the blank.

1. ____ (2)   2. ____ (7)   3. ____ (0)   4. ____ (8)
5. ____ (13)   6. ____ (47)   7. ____ (13)   8. ____ (40)
9. ____ (48)   10. ____ (12) 11. ____ (20) 12. ____ (6)
13. ____ (22) 14. ____ (4)   15. ____ (51) 16. ____ (2)
17. ____ (68) 18. ____ (13) 19. ____ (25) 20. ____ (18)
21. ____ (9)   22. ____ (27) 23. ____ (12) 24. ____ (36)
25. ____ (53) 26. ____ (5)   27. ____ (11) 28. ____ (98)
29. ____ (10) 30. ____ (7)   31. ____ (46) 32. ____ (9)
33. ____ (24) 34. ____ (1)   35. ____ (3)   36. ____ (30)
37. ____ (9)   38. ____ (50) 39. ____ (17) 40. ____ (12)
41. ____ (2)   42. ____ (95) 43. ____ (12) 44. ____ (89)
45. ____ (5)   46. ____ (7)   47. ____ (11) 48. ____ (33)
49. ____ (43) 50. ____ (20) 51. ____ (4)   52. ____ (99)
53. ____ (1)   54. ____ (9)   55. ____ (5)   56. ____ (22)
57. ____ (7)   58. ____ (0)   59. ____ (15) 60. ____ (84)
61. ____ (14) 62. ____ (8)   63. ____ (48) 64. ____ (2)
65. ____ (40) 66. ____ (14) 67. ____ (39) 68. ____ (15)
69. ____ (71) 70. ____ (2)   71. ____ (4)   72. ____ (9)
73. ____ (29) 74. ____ (9)   75. ____ (12) 76. ____ (14)
77. ____ (8)   78. ____ (3)   79. ____ (48) 80. ____ (20)
81. ____ (75) 82. ____ (43) 83. ____ (3)   84. ____ (37)

FIGURE 7.5. Example of teacher/examiner Number Identification CBM sheet. Reprinted with permission from Research Institute on Progress Monitoring.

Directions for Number Identification CBM[2]

1. Place the student copy in front of the student.
2. Place the teacher/examiner copy on the clipboard so the student cannot see it.
3. Say: **"Look at the paper in front of you. There are numbers in boxes** (point to the first box). **What number is this?"**
    a. If student gives the correct response, say: **"Good. The number is 6."** (Point to the second box.)
    b. If the student gives an incorrect response, say: **"This number is 6. What number?"** (Point to the second box.)
4. Continue with the other example(s). After the examples, turn to the first page of the student copy of the sheets.
5. Say: **"When I say begin, I want you to tell me what number is in each box. Start here and go across the page** (demonstrate by pointing). **Try each one. If you come to one that you don't know, I'll tell you what to do. Are there any questions? Put your finger on the first one. Ready? Begin."** (Trigger timer for 1 minute.)
6. On the administrator copy, write the number that the student says in the blank next to each problem number.
7. If the student comes to the end of the page, turn the page to the next page of numbers.
8. At the end of 1 minute, draw a bracket ( ]) after the last item completed and say **"Stop."**

Scoring Number Identification CBM

Submit the results using the online system. Or:

1. Count the total number of numbers attempted.
2. Count the total number of errors.
3. Calculate rate: Total items attempted – total errors = total correct per minute.
4. Calculate accuracy: total correct ÷ total items attempted = percent correct.

SCORED AS CORRECT

Number Identification CBM is scored based on each number that is stated correctly as it is associated with a correct number amount. Each correct response counts toward the total score defined as the total number correct (NC).

- Pronounced/answered correctly: The name of each number must be correctly pronounced in the correct order.
    - *Example:* 2, 10, 4, 8, 1, 12
        - Student says: 2, 10, 4, 8, 11, 12
        - Scored as: 5 NC (2, 10, 4, 8, ̸1̸, 12)

---

[2]Adapted with permission from Research Institute on Progress Monitoring.

- Self-corrections within 3 seconds: Numbers misidentified initially but corrected within 3 seconds.
  - *Example:* 8, 12, 4, 23
    - Student says: 8, 12, 23 . . . (2 sec) 4, 23
    - Scored as: 4 NC (8, 12, 4, 23)
- Dialect/articulation: Variations in pronunciation explainable by local language norms or speech sound production.
  - *Example:* 7
    - Student says: /seb-en/ instead of /sev-en/; would be accepted if this is due to an articulation problem.
    - Scored as: 1 NC
- Repetitions: Repeating the same number(s) more than once before moving on.
  - *Example:* 8, 12, 4, 23
    - Student says: 8, 12, 4 . . . 4, 23
    - Scored as: 4 NC (8, 12, 4, 23)
- Insertions: Adding numbers that are not on the stimulus sheet.
  - *Example:* 8, 12, 4, 23
    - Student says: 8, 12, 4, 86, 23 *(pointing to the appropriate number each time)*.
    - Scored as: 4 NC (8, 12, 4, 23)

SCORED AS ERRORS

All errors are marked with a slash (/).

- Mispronunciations/substitutions: When a nonnumber name or name of wrong number is given.
  - *Example:* 11
    - Student says: /oneteen/ instead of /eleven/.
    - Scored as: 0 NC (11̸)
- Omissions: Numbers that are not produced.
  - *Example:* 8, 12, 4, 23
    - Student says: 8, 12, 23
    - Scored as: 3 NC (8, 12, 4̸, 23)
- Hesitations without response: Not responding for 3 seconds and being prompted by providing the number.
  - *Example:* 8, 12, 4
    - Student says: 8, 12 . . . (3 sec). Say: ***"Try the next one."***
    - Scored as: 2 NC (8, 12, 4̸)
- Hesitations with response: Starting to respond but not finishing by 3 seconds and being prompted by providing the number.
  - *Example:* 8, 12, 4
    - Student says: 8, 12, fffffffffff (3 sec). Say: ***"Try the next one."***
    - Scored as: 2 NC (8, 12, 4̸)

- Skipped items: A number is skipped in a sequence and not stated.
  - *Example:* 8, 12, 4, 23
    - Student says: 8, 12, 23
    - Scored as: 3 NC (8, 12, 4̸, 23)

Special Administration and Scoring Considerations for Number Identification CBM

1. Correction procedure: If the student makes an error, he is not corrected. When hesitating, after 3 seconds, the student is *not* provided the correct response. The examiner should say "***Try the next one.***"
2. Skip an entire row/line: If the student skips a row of numbers, the row is crossed out and each number is counted as an error.
3. Discontinuation rule: There is no discontinuation rule for Counting CBM.
4. Finish before 1 min: If the student finishes responding before 1 minute, note the number of seconds it took to complete the sheet and prorate the score.

$$\frac{\text{Total number of NC}}{\text{Number of seconds it took to finish}} \times 60 = \text{Estimated number of NC}$$

Example: The student finished the sheet in just 50 seconds and identified 35 numbers correctly.

$$\frac{35}{50} \times 60 = 0.70 \times 60 = 42$$

We estimate that the student would have completed approximately 42 correct numbers in 1 minute had we provided more problems and timed her for the full minute.

MISSING NUMBER CBM

Missing Number CBM requires the student to identify the missing number from a pattern of four numbers in which one is replaced with a blank. This type of pattern recognition is a foundational algebraic skill as well as a demonstration of number sense and ordinality.

Materials Needed to Conduct Missing Number CBM

1. Different but equivalent stimulus sheets (student and teacher/examiner copies).
2. Directions for administering and scoring Missing Number CBM.
3. A writing utensil and clipboard or computer to enter student responses.
4. A stopwatch or countdown timer that displays seconds.
5. A quiet testing environment to work with students.
6. An equal-interval graph or a graphing program to plot the data.

Missing Number CBM Sheets

Missing Number CBM sheets should have different items. For the purposes of discussing the directions, scoring, and additional considerations we will be referring to the RIPM materials. We recommend you look at the specific measures you will be using to ensure you follow the administration and scoring rules applicable for that specific measure, as there are variations among publishers.

We recommend administering all universal screening assessments in one testing session to save setup time and for consistency in obtaining an accurate score, but it can occur across consecutive days if needed. If three samples of the same CBM task are to be administered, then the median score is used for the final score and can also be placed as the first data point on the student's graph. After that, 20–30 different but equivalent sheets will be used to monitor student progress in reading throughout the year.

Missing Number is often administered individually, but some publishers offer group administration options by having the student write the number in the blank rather than respond verbally. Two copies of the sheet will be needed. The student should have a copy of the Missing Number CBM sheet in front of him, and the teacher/examiner should either have a copy of the Missing Number sheet in front of her on the computer screen or a paper copy to write on and a writing utensil, as well as a timer and the directions. See Figures 7.6 and 7.7 for examples of each type of sheet.

Directions and Scoring Procedures for Missing Number CBM

For your convenience, Appendix B includes a reproducible version of the directions and scoring rules for Missing Number CBM.

Directions for Missing Number CBM[3]

1. Place the student copy in front of the student.
2. Place the teacher/examiner copy on the clipboard so the student cannot see it.
3. Say: *"Look at the paper in front of you. Each box has three numbers and a blank (point to the first box). What number goes in the blank?"*
   a. If student gives a correct response, say: *"Good. The number is 3."* (Point to the second box.)
   b. If the student gives an incorrect response, *"The number that goes in the blank is 3. You should have said 3 because 3 comes after 2 (0, 1, 2, 3)."* (Point to the second box).
4. Continue with the other example(s). After the examples, turn to the first page of the student copy of the sheets.
5. Say: *"When I say begin, I want you to tell me what number goes in the blank in each box. Start here and go across the page (demonstrate by pointing). Try each one. If you come to one that you don't know, I'll tell you what to do. Are there any questions? Put your finger on the first one. Ready? Begin."* (Trigger timer for 1 minute.)
6. On the administrator copy, write the number that the student says in the blank next to each problem number.

---

[3]Adapted with permission from Research Institute on Progress Monitoring.

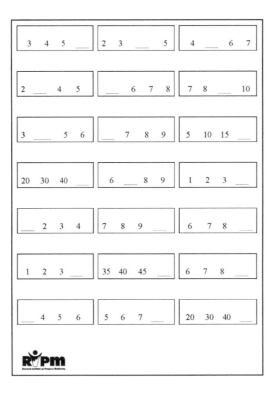

FIGURE 7.6. Example of student Missing Number CBM sheet. Reprinted with permission from Research Institute on Progress Monitoring.

Date: _____ Number Correct _____

Direction: Write the number that the student says in the blank.

1. _____ (6)	2. _____ (4)	3. _____ (5)
4. _____ (3)	5. _____ (5)	6. _____ (9)
7. _____ (4)	8. _____ (6)	9. _____ (20)
10. _____ (50)	11. _____ (7)	12. _____ (4)
13. _____ (1)	14. _____ (10)	15. _____ (9)
16. _____ (4)	17. _____ (50)	18. _____ (9)
19. _____ (3)	20. _____ (8)	21. _____ (50)
22. _____ (9)	23. _____ (8)	24. _____ (9)
25. _____ (2)	26. _____ (35)	27. _____ (30)
28. _____ (4)	29. _____ (2)	30. _____ (8)
31. _____ (3)	32. _____ (70)	33. _____ (6)
34. _____ (5)	35. _____ (10)	36. _____ (6)
37. _____ (6)	38. _____ (2)	39. _____ (4)
40. _____ (3)	41. _____ (2)	42. _____ (1)
43. _____ (2)	44. _____ (3)	45. _____ (0)
46. _____ (6)	47. _____ (50)	48. _____ (5)
49. _____ (10)	50. _____ (4)	51. _____ (40)
52. _____ (6)	53. _____ (3)	54. _____ (8)
55. _____ (4)	56. _____ (6)	57. _____ (25)
58. _____ (5)	59. _____ (90)	60. _____ (9)
61. _____ (5)	62. _____ (4)	63. _____ (1)

FIGURE 7.7. Example of teacher/examiner Missing Number CBM sheet. Reprinted with permission from Research Institute on Progress Monitoring.

7. If the student comes to the end of the page, turn the page to the next page of problems.
8. At the end of 1 minute, draw a bracket ( ]) after the last item completed and say ***"Stop."***

Scoring Missing Number CBM

Submit the results using the online system. Or:

1. Count the total number of numbers attempted.
2. Count the total number of errors.
3. Calculate rate: Total items attempted – total errors = total correct per minute.
4. Calculate accuracy: Total correct ÷ total items attempted = percent correct.

SCORED AS CORRECT

Missing Number CBM is scored based on each correct number identified that completes the number pattern. Each correct response counts toward the total score defined as the total number correct (NC).

- Pronounced/answered correctly: The name of the appropriate number to complete the pattern must be correctly pronounced.
    - *Example:* 3, 6, __, 12/ 4, 5, 6, __, / 5, __, 15, 20
        - Student says: 9, 7, 10
        - Scored as: 3 NC (9, 7, 10)
- Self-corrections within 3 seconds: Numbers misidentified initially but corrected within 3 seconds are scored as correct.
    - *Example:* 4, __, 12, 16
        - Student says: 6 (2 seconds) 8
        - Scored as: 1 NC (∅ 8)
- Dialect/articulation: Variations in pronunciation explainable by local language norms or speech sound production are correct.
    - *Example:* 10, 20, __, 40
        - Student says: /firty/ instead of /thirty/; would be accepted if this is due to an articulation problem.
        - Scored as: 1 NC (30)

SCORED AS ERRORS

All errors are marked with a slash (∕).

- Mispronunciations/substitutions: When a nonnumber name or name of wrong number is used.
    - *Example:* 2, __, 6, 8
        - Student says: /three/ instead of /four/.
        - Scored as: 0 NC (2, 4̸, 6, 8)

- Hesitations without response: Not responding for 3 seconds and being prompted by moving on to the next item.
  - *Example:* 28, 29, __, 31
    - ○ Student says: 28, 29 . . . (3 seconds). Say: "***Try the next one***."
    - ○ Scored as: 0 NC (28, 29, 3̶0̶, 31)
- Hesitations with response: Starting to respond but not finishing by 3 seconds and being prompted by moving on to the next item.
  - *Example:* 23, 26, 29, __
    - ○ Student says: thththththththth (3 seconds). Say: "***Try the next one***."
    - ○ Scored as: 0 NC (23, 26, 29, 3̶2̶)

Special Administration and Scoring Considerations for Missing Number CBM

1. Correction procedure: If the student makes an error, she is not corrected. When hesitating, after 3 seconds the student is *not* provided the correct response. The examiner should say "***Try the next one***."
2. Skip an entire row/line: If the student skips an entire row, that row is crossed out and each skipped item is an error.
3. Discontinuation rule: There is no discontinuation rule for Missing Number.
4. Finish before 1 minute: If the student finishes responding before 1 minute, his rate score should be prorated. The formula for prorating is:

$$\frac{\text{Total number of NC}}{\text{Number of seconds it took to finish}} \times 60 = \text{Estimated number of NC}$$

Example: The student finished the sheet in just 50 seconds and identified 40 numbers correctly.

$$\frac{40}{50} \times 60 = 0.8 \times 60 = 48$$

We estimate that the student would have completed approximately 48 numbers correct in 1 minute had we provided more problems and timed her for the full minute.

QUANTITY DISCRIMINATION CBM

Quantity Discrimination CBM requires the student to determine which number in a pair represents the larger quantity. Determining the relative magnitude, or size, of the quantity represented by two numbers is a component of number sense and a prerequisite skill for computation as well as problem solving.

Materials Needed to Conduct Quantity Discrimination

1. Different but equivalent stimulus sheets (student and teacher/examiner copies).
2. Directions for administering and scoring Quantity Discrimination.
3. A writing utensil and clipboard or computer to enter student responses.
4. A stopwatch or countdown timer that displays seconds.
5. A quiet testing environment to work with students.
6. An equal-interval graph or a graphing program to plot the data.

Quantity Discrimination CBM Sheets

Quantity Discrimination CBM sheets should have different items. For the purposes of discussing the directions, scoring, and additional considerations we will be referring to the RIPM materials. We recommend you look at the specific measures you will be using to ensure you follow the administration and scoring rules applicable for that specific measure, as there are variations among publishers.

We recommend administering all universal screening assessments in one testing session to save setup time and for consistency in obtaining an accurate score, but it can occur across consecutive days if needed. If three samples of the same CBM task are to be administered, then the median score is used for the final score and can also be placed as the first data point on the student's graph. After that, 20–30 different but equivalent sheets will be used to monitor student progress in reading throughout the year.

Quantity Discrimination CBM is often administered individually, but some publishers offer group administration options by having the student circle the number that represents the larger quantity rather than respond verbally. Two copies of the sheet will be needed. The student should have a copy of the Quantity Discrimination CBM sheet in front of him, and the teacher/examiner should have either a copy of the Quantity Discrimination CBM sheet in front of her on the computer screen or a paper copy to write on and a writing utensil, as well as a timer and the directions. See Figures 7.8 and 7.9 for examples of each type of sheet.

Directions and Scoring Procedures for Quantity Discrimination CBM

For your convenience, Appendix B includes a reproducible version of the directions and scoring rules for Quantity Discrimination.

Directions for Quantity Discrimination CBM[4]

1. Place the student copy in front of the student.
2. Place the teacher/examiner copy on the clipboard so the student cannot see it.

---

[4]Adapted with permission from Research Institute on Progress Monitoring.

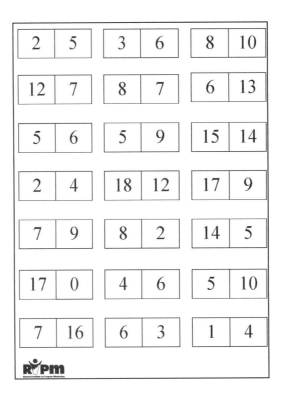

2	5		3	6		8	10
12	7		8	7		6	13
5	6		5	9		15	14
2	4		18	12		17	9
7	9		8	2		14	5
17	0		4	6		5	10
7	16		6	3		1	4

FIGURE 7.8. Example of student Quantity Discrimination CBM sheet. Reprinted with permission from Research Institute on Progress Monitoring.

Date: _____   Number Correct _____

Direction: Write the number that the student says in the blank.

1. _____ (5)   2. _____ (6)   3. _____ (10)
4. _____ (12)   5. _____ (8)   6. _____ (13)
7. _____ (6)   8. _____ (9)   9. _____ (15)
10. _____ (4)   11. _____ (18) 12. _____ (17)
13. _____ (9)   14. _____ (8)   15. _____ (14)
16. _____ (17) 17. _____ (6)   18. _____ (10)
19. _____ (16) 20. _____ (6)   21. _____ (4)
22. _____ (16) 23. _____ (6)   24. _____ (9)
25. _____ (6)   26. _____ (18) 27. _____ (5)
28. _____ (7)   29. _____ (20) 30. _____ (4)
31. _____ (5)   32. _____ (10) 33. _____ (17)
34. _____ (5)   35. _____ (17) 36. _____ (10)
37. _____ (17) 38. _____ (6)   39. _____ (13)
40. _____ (5)   41. _____ (16) 42. _____ (9)
43. _____ (8)   44. _____ (10) 45. _____ (11)
46. _____ (9)   47. _____ (17) 48. _____ (3)
49. _____ (4)   50. _____ (13) 51. _____ (8)
52. _____ (14) 53. _____ (8)   54. _____ (3)
55. _____ (9)   56. _____ (17) 57. _____ (13)
58. _____ (8)   59. _____ (5)   60. _____ (20)
61. _____ (5)   62. _____ (13) 63. _____ (10)

FIGURE 7.9. Example of teacher/examiner Quantity Discrimination CBM sheet. Reprinted with permission from Research Institute on Progress Monitoring.

3. Say: *"Look at the paper in front of you. In each row there are some boxes with numbers in them"* (point to the first box). *"I want you to tell me the number that is bigger."*
   a. If the student gives the correct response, say: *"Good. 7 is bigger than 1."* (Point to the second box.)
   b. If the student gives an incorrect response, say: *"The number that is bigger is 7. You should have said 7 because 7 is bigger than 1."* (Point to the second box.)
4. Continue with the other example(s). After the examples, turn to the first page of the student copy of the sheets.
5. Say: *"When I say begin, I want you to tell me which number is bigger. Start here and go across the page (demonstrate by pointing). Try each one. If you come to one that you don't know, I'll tell you what to do. Are there any questions? Put your finger on the first one. Ready? Begin."* (Trigger timer for 1 minute.)
6. On the administrator copy, write the number that the student says in the blank next to each problem number.
7. If the student comes to the end of the page, turn the page to the next page of problems.
8. At the end of 1 minute, draw a bracket ( ]) after the last item completed and say *"Stop."*

Scoring Quantity Discrimination CBM

Submit the results using the online system. Or:

1. Count the total number of numbers attempted.
2. Count the total number of errors.
3. Calculate rate: Total items attempted – total errors = total correct per minute.
4. Calculate accuracy: Total correct ÷ total items attempted = percent correct.

SCORED AS CORRECT

Quantity Discrimination CBM is scored based on each correct response the student gives that indicates the bigger number. Each correct response counts toward the total score defined as the total number correct (NC).

- Pronounced/answered correctly: The name of the appropriate larger number must be correctly pronounced.
  - *Example:* [2 | 8] [6 | 4] [3 | 1]
    - Student says: 8, 6, 3
    - Scored as: 3 NC (8, 6, 3)
- Self-corrections within 3 seconds: Numbers misidentified initially but corrected within 3 seconds.
  - *Example:* [5 | 6]
    - Student says: 5 (2 seconds) 6
    - Scored as: 1 NC (6)
- Dialect/articulation: Variations in pronunciation explainable by local language norms or speech sound production.

- *Example:* [7 | 4]
  - o Student says: /seb-en/ instead of /sev-en/; would be accepted if this is due to an articulation problem.
  - o Scored as: 1 NC (7)

SCORED AS ERRORS

All errors are marked with a slash (╱).

- Mispronunciations/substitutions: When a nonnumber name or name of a wrong number is used.
  - *Example:* [11 | 10]
    - o Student says: /oneteen/ instead of /eleven/.
    - o Scored as: 0 NC (11̸)
- Hesitations without response: Not responding for 3 seconds and being prompted to move to the next item.
  - *Example:* [21 | 23] [8 | 10]
    - o Student says: 23 (3 seconds). Say: ***"Try the next one."***
    - o Scored as: 1 NC (23, 1̸0̸)
- Hesitations with response: Starting to respond but not finishing by 3 seconds and being prompted to move to the next item.
  - *Example:* [5 | 3]
    - o Student says: fffffffffff (3 seconds). Say: ***"Try the next one."***
    - o Scored as: 0 NC (3̸)
- Skipped items: A number that is skipped in a sequence.
  - *Example:* [29 | 26] [8 | 9] [14 | 12]
    - o Student says: 29, 14
    - o Scored as: 2 NC (29, ∅̸, 14)

Special Administration and Scoring Considerations for Quantity Discrimination CBM

1. Correction procedure: If the student makes an error, he is not corrected. When hesitating, after 3 seconds the student is *not* provided the correct response. The examiner should say ***"Try the next one."***
2. Skip an entire row/line: If the student skips an entire row, that row is crossed out and each skipped item is an error.
3. Discontinuation rule: There is no discontinuation rule for Quantity Discrimination.
4. Finish before 1 minute: If the student finishes responding before 1 minute, his rate score should be prorated. The formula for prorating is:

$$\frac{\text{Total number of NC}}{\text{Number of seconds it took to finish}} \times 60 = \text{Estimated number of NC}$$

Example: The student finished the sheet in just 50 seconds and identified 35 numbers correctly.

$$\frac{35}{50} \times 60 = 0.70 \times 60 = 42$$

We estimate that the student would have completed approximately 42 numbers correct in 1 minute had we provided more problems and timed him for the full minute.

HOW OFTEN SHOULD EARLY NUMERACY CBM BE ADMINISTERED?

In Chapter 2, we provide additional details on how often and when to administer CBM for the different purposes of universal screening and progress monitoring. Below we provide only an outline for these purposes. We suggest you refer to Chapter 2 for a more in-depth discussion on how often and when to give CBM for these different purposes.

Universal Screening

All students should be screened using grade level materials three times a year. This typically occurs in fall, winter, and spring. Universal screening data assist in answering some important questions, two of which are:

"Is this student *at risk* for academic failure by the end of the year?"
"Is our core instruction meeting the needs of most of our students?"

Progress Monitoring

Only those students who have been identified as *at risk*, meaning he did not score at or above the benchmark score on the universal screening assessment, should be progress monitored at least once a week on instructional level material and at least once per month on grade level materials if it is different from instructional level. An important aspect of progress monitoring is to do it often (i.e., weekly) and consistently (i.e., using CBM materials that are at the same difficulty level). Progress monitoring data assist in answering two very important questions:

"Is this student benefiting from the instruction she is receiving?"
"Is this intervention helping the majority of the students who have received it?"

HOW MUCH TIME DOES IT TAKE
TO ADMINISTER AND SCORE EARLY NUMERACY CBM?

The time needed to score each student sheet is the same for Counting CBM, Number Identification CBM, Missing Number CBM, and Quantity Discrimination CBM. Once the student is in front of the teacher/examiner, the time it takes to give the directions, have the student do the task for 1 minute, and score the sheet is 2–3 minutes total. If you are universally screening and giving three sheets at one time it should take 5–6 minutes total. You will also need to factor in time for the student to move to where the teacher/examiner is, whether that is in the same room or down the hall. Obviously, it makes more sense to go to the students rather than have the students come to the examiner as one way to save time. Another way to save time is to have everything printed out and ready to go with the students' names already indicated on the appropriate forms. One way to do this is to print labels.

EARLY NUMERACY CBM SCORES

There is currently no research on benchmarks for any of the early numeracy curriculum-based measures (aimsweb publishes "default cut scores," but these are norms using the 35th and 15th percentiles rather than empirically derived cut scores). If you remember from Chapter 2, we indicated that benchmarks are helpful because they are predictive of later student achievement. This allows teachers to determine who is on track and who needs additional assistance to be successful in early numeracy and, in turn, math.

In the absence of empirically derived benchmarks, norms for Early Numeracy CBM are the best currently available option. The norms are helpful because they provide a way of comparing a student's score to the performance of others in her grade or at her instructional level. The norms can then be used to determine how much growth we would expect the student to make to either maintain her level of relative performance or close the gap between her performance and her peers'. Table 7.1 provides information on norms for Early Numeracy CBM for kindergarten and grade 1.

HOW DO I USE THE INFORMATION
TO WRITE EARLY NUMERACY IEP GOALS AND OBJECTIVES?

Writing goals and objectives is a helpful way to define the behavior of interest and how it will be measured in order to be able to make decisions about a students learning. Chapter 2 provides the seven steps needed to write a good goal or objective. The seven steps include: time, learner, behavior, level, content, material, and criteria. Here, we will provide only an example for Counting CBM but we encourage you to look at Chapter 2 for further information.

TABLE 7.1. Norms for Early Numeracy CBM

	Kindergarten			Grade 1		
Percentile	Fall	Winter	Spring	Fall	Winter	Spring
	Oral Counting (correct oral counts)					
90%	70	91	100	96	—	—
75%	57	78	91	84	98	100
50%	**39**	**64**	**78**	**72**	**86**	**94**
25%	26	49	64	59	73	80
10%	14	39	49	46	61	69
	Number Identification (correct number identifications)					
90%	56	—	—	63	80	80
75%	47	56	—	54	72	77
50%	**33**	**52**	**56**	**43**	**61**	**66**
25%	15	39	51	30	50	56
10%	4	25	40	17	39	45
	Missing Number (correct missing number)					
90%	15	21	—	20	26	28
75%	10	17	20	16	22	24
50%	**5**	**12**	**16**	**12**	**18**	**21**
25%	1	7	11	7	14	16
10%	0	3	7	3	10	12
	Quantity Discrimination (correct quantity discriminations)					
90%	26	—	—	34	40	—
75%	19	28	28	28	38	40
50%	**11**	**21**	**28**	**22**	**32**	**36**
25%	5	12	22	14	26	30
10%	1	6	12	6	18	24

Note. Data from aimsweb (2015).

Example of Goal

- Counting goal
  - In 30 weeks, Larry will count circles from a kindergarten math touch counting Early Numeracy CBM sheet at 50 NC in 1 minute with greater than 95% accuracy.

The same principles apply when writing objectives, but one should use a shorter time frame.

Example of Objective

- Counting objective
  - In 10 weeks, Larry will count circles from a kindergarten math touch counting Early Numeracy CBM sheet at 20 NC in 1 minute with greater than 95% accuracy.

FREQUENTLY ASKED QUESTIONS ABOUT EARLY NUMERACY CBM

1. *Do teachers generally administer Early Numeracy CBM sheets one-on-one with each student or to a group?* Most early numeracy curriculum-based measures need to be administered individually because they require a verbal response. However, there have been some researchers who have experimented with group administration for missing numbers and quantity discrimination by having the students write their responses or circle the larger number. When universally screening a whole class, it might make sense to administer to the entire group. When doing weekly progress monitoring, we recommend individual administration.

2. *My student has improved her math performance as I have monitored her progress, but she is not receiving any instruction in math. Could assessment using CBM alone be making a difference?* The extra 1 minute of "practice" that she is getting per week is probably not enough to cause improvement. She may be practicing elsewhere or receiving additional instruction.

3. *I only have 20 Early Numeracy CBM sheets, but I need to progress monitor for 35 weeks. Is it OK to use the same sheets again?* Yes. Once you have used all 20, start using them again. The student probably doesn't remember specific items she did 20 weeks ago. This also means that you should not use the sheets as homework or additional practice. The Early Numeracy CBM tasks are not ones you want to provide instruction in directly; they are skills that are good indicators of performance.

4. *Because there are no benchmark scores on early numeracy curriculum-based measures, can I use norms to put students in instructional groups?* Yes, if you have students with similar instructional needs. These groups should be flexible and students should be evaluated and regrouped every 6–8 weeks.

5. *Not everyone in my class is on the same instructional level. Should I still give them all the same Early Numeracy CBM sheets?* All students should be screened on their grade-level skills, but they should be progress monitored on their instructional level, especially if they are receiving instruction on that level. Early Numeracy CBM is most appropriate for grades K–1, but instruction for students in grades 2 and above who are struggling might include skills that are important for that student to master. The best way to handle this is to give both the grade-level and the instructional-level measures each week so that you have an indication of how students are doing given the instruction they are receiving (instructional level) and how well it is transferring to more complex problems or skills (grade level).

6. *What should I do with the scored sheets?* This information can be kept in a portfolio along with the graphed data to demonstrate progress over the year.

RESOURCES AND/OR FURTHER READING

Chard, D., Clarke, B., Baker, S., Otterstedt, J., Braun, D., & Katz, R. (2005). Using measures of number sense to screen for difficulties in mathematics: Preliminary findings. *Assessment for Effective Intervention, 30*(2), 3–14.

Clarke, B., & Shinn, M. (2004). A preliminary investigation into the identification and development of early mathematics curriculum-based measurement. *School Psychology Review, 33,* 234–248.

Hampton, D., Lembke, E., Lee, Y-S., Pappas, S., Chiong, C., & Ginsburg, H. (2011). Technical adequacy of early numeracy curriculum-based measures for kindergarten and first-grade students. *Assessment for Effective Intervention, 36,* 118–126.

Hojnoski, R., Silberglitt, B., & Floyd, R. (2009). Sensitivity to growth over time of the preschool numeracy indicators with a sample of preschoolers in head start. *School Psychology Review, 38,* 402–418.

Methe, S., Begeny, J., & Leary, L. (2011). Development of conceptually focused early numeracy skill indicators. *Assessment for Effective Intervention, 36,* 230–242.

Methe, S., Hojnoski, R., Clarke, B., Owens, B., Lilley, P., Politoylo, B., et al. (2011). Innovations and future directions for early numeracy curriculum-based measurement: Commentary on the Special Series. *Assessment for Effective Intervention, 36,* 200–209.

CHAPTER 8

How to Conduct Math CBM

WHY SHOULD I CONDUCT MATH CBM?

Reading and literacy are often considered the most important skills taught in schools; however, many argue that math is similarly important for success in life. Just as for other skills, Math CBM provides a reliable and valid way to identify (1) students who are at risk for failure, (2) students who are not making adequate progress given the instruction they are receiving, (3) students who need additional diagnostic evaluation, and (4) students' instructional level. Most math assessments do not provide information about automaticity, which is just as big a drawback as it is for reading since automaticity provides information about skill mastery.

Math CBM is easy and efficient to administer and score. It can be administered individually or to an entire class at the same time. Math CBM can be broken down into three areas: early numeracy, computation, and concepts and applications. Early Numeracy CBM was already the focus of Chapter 7, so this chapter will focus on Computation (M-COMP) CBM and Concepts and Applications (M-CAP) CBM. M-COMP CBM was the original approach to CBM in math developed in the early 1980s and, as such, has the most research to support its use. It was used because of the need for a quick and easy method to measure computation performance that would be reliable and relate to outcome measures.

M-COMP CBM

Computation is a foundational component to mathematics. Automaticity with computation is required to facilitate problem solving and application of math reasoning skills.

Materials Needed to Conduct M-COMP CBM

1. Different but equivalent math sheets (student and teacher/examiner copies).
2. Directions for administering and scoring M-COMP CBM.
3. A writing utensil for the student or computer to enter student responses.
4. A writing utensil and clipboard for the teacher/examiner.
5. A stopwatch or countdown timer that displays seconds.
6. A quiet testing environment to work with students.
7. An equal-interval graph or a graphing program to plot the data.

M-COMP CBM Sheets

Other content areas such as reading or writing generally allow for generic passages, lists, or story starters. For example, reading passages at a third-grade level of complexity are pretty similar regardless of curriculum. Math, however, has a more specific scope and sequence. M-COMP CBM is conducted by having the student answer computational problems for 2 minutes (or more as determined by grade level and publisher). The teacher/examiner then counts the number of correct digits (CD) that the student computed. Notice that this is not correct problems, like many other math assessments use, but correct digits. We'll discuss why in the section on scoring. More importantly, the information gathered provides a database for each student so that appropriate instructional decisions can be made in a timely manner. Although this can vary from state to state, school to school, and curriculum to curriculum, with recent advances by the National Mathematics Advisory Panel (2008) and National Council for Teachers of Mathematics (2000), and the Common Core State Standards (National Governors Association Center for Best Practices & Council of Chief State School Officers, 2010), there is a convergence of the content associated with each grade level. Most educators like to have math sheets that are linked directly to the skills included in their state's core curriculum (Why wouldn't you want to have your progress monitoring measure aligned with the outcome measure used at the end of the year?). As such, generic or premade sheets may not include the same skills at each level. If you cannot find premade sheets that fit your curriculum (see Box 8.1 for information on where to obtain some), here is a guide for creating your own. It can also serve as a reference for judging the utility of other sheets you may consider purchasing. Creating your own sheets is more time consuming, but once it is done, you have a great and useful set of materials. To cut the workload, try to find others who can make some of the sheets for the grade level or even do some of the other grades. You can also go to one of many websites (listed in the "Resources and/or Further Reading" section at the end of this chapter) that will help you create M-COMP CBM sheets.

The math tests used for universal screening and progress monitoring usually take the form of SBMs. As you will recall from Chapter 1, SBMs consist of the specific skills expected to be mastered by the end of the year rather than a general, capstone task such as those used in GOMs (which is what has been presented for Reading and Writing CBMs in the previous chapters). The math sheets themselves should have different problems but be equivalent in complexity (i.e., at the same grade level) and should have at least 25 problems per page

---

BOX 8.1. Where to Find Premade Math CBM Sheets

$ indicates there is a cost for the materials and/or graphing program.
⌨ indicates computerized administration available.
✎ indicates data management and graphing available.

aimsweb (Pearson) $✎

Website: *www.aimsweb.com*

Phone: 866-313-6194

Products: • Computation
          • Concepts and Applications

Easy CBM $✎

Website: *www.easycbm.com*

Phone: 800-323-9540

Products: • Numbers and Operations
          • Geometry
          • Numbers Operations and Algebra

Edcheckup $✎

Website: *www.edcheckup.com*

Phone: 612-454-0074

Products: • Cloze Math

FastBridge Learning $⌨✎

Website: *www.fastbridge.org*

Phone: 612-424-3714

Products: • Computation

mCLASS: Math $⌨✎

Website: *www.amplify.com*

Phone: 800-823-1969

Products: • Computation
          • Concepts and Applications

MBSP Basic Math Computation—Second Edition (PRO-ED) $

Website: *www.proedinc.com/customer/productView.aspx?ID=1431*

Phone: 800-897-3202

Products: • Computation
          • Concepts and Applications

System to Enhance Educational Performance (STEEP) $✎

Website: *www.isteep.com*

Phone: 800-881-9142

Products: • Computation
          • Concepts and Applications

(continued)

> **Vanderbilt University $ (copying, postage, and handling only)**
>
> Website: *www.peerassistedlearningstrategies.com*
>
> Phone: 615-343-4782
>
> E-mail: *lynn.a.davies@vanderbilt.edu*
>
> Products: • Computation
>   • Concepts and Applications

(Fuchs & Fuchs, 1991; see Figure 8.1).[1] The math problems should represent the skills the student is expected to master throughout the entire school year. This is accomplished by examining the yearlong math curriculum and determining the emphasis on the skills covered during the year. Based on which skills will be taught and how much time is spent teaching each skill (an indicator of emphasis), math problems are selected or developed for each sheet. While the problems on each sheet should have different numerals (i.e., problems testing the same skill should contain different numbers), the number of problems represent-

---

Math: Grade 3   Sheet 1

Name: _____   Date: _____

6 × 7	952 + 768	614 − 44	156 + 32	141 − 30
476 − 143	9 × 0	156 + 284	982 − 97	321 + 147
241 + 118	829 − 106	6 × 0	86 + 78	328 − 142
41 −18	564 + 222	98 − 17	9 × 5	249 + 92
409 + 292	728 − 260	311 + 188	256 − 45	4 × 1

FIGURE 8.1. Example of student mixed-operation M-COMP CBM sheet.

---

[1]Some people use the common rule that fluency sheets should contain 30–40% more items (in this case digits, not problems) than the criterion for acceptable performance (CAP). This way if a student finishes the sheet, you know that she is performing well above the CAP anyway and there is not a concern about her performance. For example, mastery level (i.e., the CAP) for fourth grade is greater than 49 CD. If your fluency sheet contains at least 64–69 digits, any student who finishes the sheet accurately in less than 2 minutes is probably doing fine.

ing each skill should be the same on every sheet. Therefore, each sheet is equivalent and represents the curriculum from the entire year (Fuchs & Fuchs, 1991).

For example, a third-grade curriculum might include the following math computation skills:

1. Multidigit addition without regrouping.
2. Multidigit addition with regrouping.
3. Multidigit subtraction without regrouping.
4. Multidigit subtraction with regrouping.
5. Multiplication facts, factors to 9.

If these skills appear to be equally weighted in the curriculum, we include an equal number of items for each skill on each sheet. This gives us a 5×5 grid to guide the construction of the 25-item sheet. Figure 8.1 is an example of what one of our third-grade math sheets might look like. Skills-based sheets such as the one in Figure 8.1 are sometimes called mixed-operation sheets because they contain problems requiring different math computation skills that are included in the year's curriculum.

Notice that the items on the sheet are not in the order in which they are presented in the curriculum (i.e., multidigit addition without regrouping first, multiplication facts last). The order of the items is random so that they are not in order of increasing complexity, but they are in a systematic order after the first line. Looking down the sheet, you can see that similar item types are grouped diagonally. This can assist us when looking for patterns in student responses to specific types of math problems. Making plans at this stage helps provide us with valuable information when using the sheets. We will discuss this in more detail later in the chapter.

Another way to create math sheets is to create sheets that test only one operation (see Figure 8.2). Single-operation math sheets should contain only problems involving one operation. A single-operation sheet can be created using only the basic facts of that operation (e.g., addition facts of addends 0–9, sums 0–18 as in Figure 8.2). When a student is just beginning to learn an operation, this type of sheet can be helpful for short-term planning. A single-operation sheet can also be created using a combination of within-operation skills. For example, the sheet could contain basic facts, 2 digit × 2 digit addition without regrouping, 2 digit × 2 digit addition with regrouping, 3 digit × 3 digit addition without regrouping, 3 digit × 3 digit addition with regrouping, and so forth. This type of sheet isn't appropriate for universal screening or progress monitoring (because it only assesses one skill), but it can be used to gain some diagnostic information or to use as a starting point for a CBE approach to decision making (Hosp et al., 2014).

Two copies of each math sheet will be needed: one copy for the student to write on (Figure 8.1 is an example) and one copy for the teacher/examiner that contains the correct answers and indicates the correct number of digits for each problem (see Figure 8.3). A correct digit is the right numeral in the right place (see "Directions and Scoring Procedures for Math CBM" below for specific guidelines).

We recommend administering all universal screening assessments in one testing session to save setup time and for consistency in obtaining an accurate score, but it can occur

Math: Addition Facts

Name: _____   Date: _____

9 + 3	1 + 3	1 + 6	3 + 8	1 + 6
2 + 1	1 + 8	4 + 7	6 + 8	5 + 2
2 + 6	8 + 8	2 + 7	3 + 3	3 + 4
1 + 1	5 + 2	8 + 1	8 + 7	9 + 1
8 + 2	1 + 8	2 + 3	6 + 5	1 + 5

FIGURE 8.2. Example of teacher/examiner single-operation M-COMP CBM sheet.

across consecutive days if needed. If three samples of the same assessment are to be administered, then the median score is used for the final score and can also be placed as the first data point on the student's graph. After that, 20–30 different but equivalent sheets will be used to monitor student progress in math throughout the year.

M-COMP CBM can be administered individually or to a group. Two copies of the sheet will be needed. The student should have a pencil or pen and a copy of the M-COMP CBM sheet in front of him, and the teacher/examiner should have either a copy of the M-COMP CBM sheet in front of her on the computer screen or a paper copy to write on and a writing utensil, as well as a timer and the directions. See Figures 8.1 and 8.3 for examples of each type of sheet.

Directions and Scoring Procedures for M-COMP CBM

For your convenience, Appendix B includes a reproducible version of the directions and scoring rules for M-COMP CBM.

Directions for M-COMP CBM[2]

1. Place a copy of the student sheet in front of the students.
2. For single-operation sheets, say: ***"The sheets on your desk have*** (*addition, subtraction,*

---

[2]Adapted with permission from Shinn (1989).

multiplication, division, fractions, ratios, decimals, etc.) **problems on them. Look at each problem carefully before you answer it. When I say, 'Please begin,' start answering the problems. Begin with the first problem and work across the page** (*point*). **Then go to the next row. If you cannot answer the problem, mark an 'X' through it and go to the next one. If you finish a page, turn the page and continue working until I say 'Thank you.' Are there any questions? Please begin."**

For mixed-operation sheets, say: **"The sheets on your desk have math problems on them. There are several types of problems on the sheet. Some are** (*insert types of problems on sheet*). **Look at each problem carefully before you answer it. When I say 'Please begin,' start answering the problems. Begin with the first problem and work across the page** (*point*). **Then go to the next row. If you cannot answer the problem, mark an 'X' through it and go to the next one. If you finish a page, turn the page and continue working until I say 'Thank you.' Are there any questions? Please begin."**

3. Once you say **"Please begin,"** start the countdown timer (*set for 2 minutes or the appropriate time limit*). At the end of the time limit, say **"Thank you"** and have the students put their pencils down and stop working.

Math: Grade 3   Sheet 1

Name: _____   Date: _____

6	952	614	156	141	
× 7	+ 768	− 44	+ 32	−30	
42	**1720**	**570**	**188**	**111**	15(15)
(2)	(4)	(3)	(3)	(3)	
476	9	156	982	321	
−143	× 0	+ 284	− 97	+ 147	
333	**0**	**440**	**885**	**468**	13(28)
(3)	(1)	(3)	(3)	(3)	
241	829	6	86	328	
+ 118	− 106	× 0	+ 78	−142	
359	**723**	**0**	**164**	**186**	13(41)
(3)	(3)	(1)	(3)	(3)	
41	564	98	9	249	
− 18	+ 222	− 17	× 5	+ 92	
23	**786**	**81**	**45**	**341**	12(53)
(2)	(3)	(2)	(2)	(3)	
409	728	311	256	4	
+ 292	− 260	+ 188	− 45	× 1	
701	**468**	**499**	**211**	**4**	13(66)
(3)	(3)	(3)	(3)	(1)	

FIGURE 8.3. Example of teacher/examiner mixed-operation M-COMP CBM sheet.

Scoring M-COMP CBM

Submit the results using the online system. Or:

1. Count the total number attempted.
2. Count the total number of errors.
3. Calculate rate: Total items attempted – total errors = total correct per time (2–8 minutes).
4. Calculate accuracy: Total correct ÷ total items attempted = percent correct.

When scoring M-COMP CBM, there are actually three ways that publishers are now recommending. First, as originally developed, the number of correct digits in the solution (CD-S) to the problem (which includes critical processes, not just the answer), rather than the number of correct problems was used because it is a more sensitive measure to change. It is also considered a fairer metric because the student is awarded more points for correctly solving more complex problems. Since complex problems generally take more time to solve than basic ones, a greater number of points is available for the greater time commitment (this is important on a timed task). This is a simple way of weighting the complexity of computation problems.

Second, some M-COMP CBM programs only count the total number of correct digits in the answer (CD-A). This may be problematic because a division problem that has three CD-A would be worth the same number of points as an addition problem with three CD-A despite the additional steps (i.e., critical processes). However, it makes scoring easier and more reliable.

Third, some M-COMP CBM programs are including calculation of correct problems (CP). Although this metric is not as sensitive to growth as CD, it does have good generalizability because ultimately it is important for the student to get the entire problem correct. It might be a better metric for universal screening rather than progress monitoring, but more research is needed.

Some publishers are exploring additional ways of weighting problems for the amount of time it typically takes to compute the answer in relation to the number of CD or CP awarded. The most common method seems to be assigning each problem between one and three points for a correct answer and none for an incorrect answer. When comparing your students' performance to the publisher's benchmarks or norms, it is crucial to use the same scoring metric, CD-S, CD-A, and/or CP, as those used to develop the benchmarks or norms.

Figure 8.4 shows two math problems. If we were counting the number of *problems* correct, each would be worth one point. When counting the number of *digits* correct, a correct answer for the first problem (see panel A) would be worth 2 CD because that is how many are included in the longest approach to solve that problem. This would be the same for both CD-S and CD-A. If a student got one of those digits wrong (e.g., wrote 40 instead of 41—see panel D), she would get credit for one digit rather than no credit for the problem.

In the second example, there are 21 digits in the long version of solving the problem and 6 digits in the correct answer (see panel B). This is where CD-S and CD-A differ. If the student got the correct answer, she would get 6 CD-A (for 182,928), but 21 CD-S (because of the intermediary critical processes). If the student did all the steps correctly except for

A	B	C
25 + 16 **41**	1236 x 148 **9888** **49440** **123600** **182928**	1236 x 148 **182928**
2 CD-S 2 CD-A 1 CP	21 CD-S 6 CD-A 1 CP	21 CD-S 6 CD-A 1 CP
D	E	F
25 + 16 4Ø	1236 x 148 **9888** **49440** **123600** **182828**	1236 x 148 182828
1 CD-S 1 CD-A 0 CP	20 CD-S 5 CD-A 0 CP	5 CD-S 5 CD-A 0 CP

FIGURE 8.4. Sample math problems with correct problems and digits.

one and got an answer of 182,828 (rather than 182,928), she would get credit for 5 CD-A or 20 CD-S (panel E). When a student makes an error in one step of a multistep solution (e.g., the second problem in Figure 8.4 has a transcription error in the answer—the student wrote 8 instead of 9 even though she did all the work correctly), the scoring really differs. If the scoring were by problem, she would get no credit. If the scoring is by digit, she is only penalized for the one digit that is incorrect. For the example in Figure 8.4, this holds true for both CD-S and CD-A. However, for a student who does not show her work (see panels C and F), her CD-S and CD-A would be equal. CD-S and CD-A only differ for multistep problems where the student makes an error in the answer. Also note that CP is equal at zero for all three types of responses because they all include at least one incorrect digit.

For each M-COMP problem, the number of correct digits is counted and then they are added together to get the total number of CD. For the student to get credit for a CD it must be the right digit in the right place.

SCORED AS CORRECT

- Answered correctly: If the student has the correct answer, she is given credit for 1 CP, the number of CD in the answer (CD-A), or the longest method used to solve the problem *even if all the work is not shown* (for CD-S). If the student gets the correct answer, she has demonstrated that she knows how to solve the problem and, therefore, gets full credit in whichever metric is used.

- Incomplete/crossed out: If a problem has been crossed out or started, but not completed, the student still receives appropriate credit. Correct work is correct work, even if the student did not finish the problem.

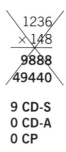

9 CD-S
0 CD-A
0 CP

- Reversed/rotated: Reversed or rotated digits are scored as correct with the exception of 6's and 9's. With 6's and 9's, it is not possible to tell which one the student meant to write. No other digits can become others through rotation or reversal.

25	25
+ 16	+ 16
41	∌1
2 CD-S	**2 CD-S**
2 CD-A	**2 CD-A**
1 CP	**1 CP**

- Placeholder: In multiplication problems, any symbol used as a placeholder is counted as a correct digit as long as it is holding a place that needs to be held. The student can use a 0, X, ☺, a blank space, or whatever else as long as it is used to hold that place.

1236	1236
× 148	× 148
9888	9888
49440	4944x
123600	123600
182928	182928
21 CD-S	**21 CD-S**
6 CD-A	**6 CD-A**
1 CP	**1 CP**

SCORED AS ERRORS

All errors are marked with a slash (/). See Figure 8.4 (panels D, E, and F) for three examples.

- Substitutions: When the student writes the wrong number.
- Omissions: Each number omitted is an error.

Special Administration and Scoring Considerations for M-COMP CBM

1. Correction procedure: If the student makes an error, he is *not* corrected. Particularly because M-COMP CBM can be administered to a group, error correction is not possible or appropriate.

2. Skip an entire row/line: If a student skips an entire row that row is not included in the scoring. Because of the curriculum-sampling nature of M-COMP CBM, a student might not be able to complete the problems in a row. If this is the case, that is OK; however, it is important to check the student's work to ensure that he is attempting problems you know he has been exposed to in order to determine his skill with the task.

3. Finish before time limit: If the student finishes in less than 2 minutes, note the number of seconds it took to complete the math sheet and prorate the score. The formula for prorating is:

$$\frac{\text{Total number of CD}}{\text{Number of seconds it took to finish}} \times 120 = \text{Estimated number of CD}$$

Example: The student finished the math sheet in just 110 seconds and got 40 digits correct.

$$\frac{40}{110} \times 120 = 43.6$$

We estimate that the student would have completed approximately 44 correct digits in 2 minutes had we provided more problems and timed her for the full 2 minutes.

Prorating is only appropriate for CD-S and CD-A because they are designed to be more sensitive measures to growth. Another consideration is publishers' materials that now require 4, 8, or 10 minutes for M-COMP CBM. These are designed to make it less likely that the student will complete the sheets in the allotted time.

4. Answers above the line: If the student writes parts of the answer above the line, as with carrying or borrowing, they are not counted as correct digits. These are part of the work of the solution—not the solution itself—and their correctness is shown in the answer below the line.

```
                                    1 2 4
        1236                     1236
      × 148                    × 148
        9888                     9888
       49440                    49440
      123600                   123600
      182928                   182928

      21 CD-S                  21 CD-S
       6 CD-A                   6 CD-A
       1 CP                     1 CP
```

5. In division, a basic fact is when both the divisor and the quotient are 9 or less. For the purposes of scoring, the total CD is always 1. Also, remainders of 0 are not counted as correct digits nor are placeholders; therefore, they are not included in the scoring.

$$8\overline{)24} \quad\quad 3\overline{)9}$$
$$\phantom{8\overline{)}}3 \quad\quad\phantom{3\overline{)}}3$$

M-CAP CBM

A problem many people have with using M-COMP CBM as the sole skill measured by Math CBM is that, especially in the older grades, there is a lot more to math than computation. Therefore, Math CBM has been extended to include other math skills. M-CAP includes other math skills such as measurement, time, graph interpretation, and many others found in math curriculums. M-CAP CBM measures deviate from traditional Math CBM in a few ways. First, the response format may vary—some are fill in the blank; others are multiple choice. Second, when used with lower-grade students, the measure is read to the student, but all others complete it independently. Reading the measure to the students attempts to reduce the effect of reading skills on the student's performance. Third, the time limit provided is 6–10 minutes, typically longer than for M-COMP CBM or Early Numeracy CBM. Because the skills are more complex and varied, extra time is needed; however, this does make use of the measure more time consuming.

M-CAP CBM is conducted by having the student answer math problems for 8–10 minutes (as determined by grade level and publisher). The teacher/examiner then counts the number of problems that the student answered correctly and assigns the appropriate number of points for each problem according to the answer key.

Materials Needed to Conduct M-CAP CBM

1. Different but equivalent math sheets (student and teacher/examiner copies).
2. Directions for administering and scoring M-CAP CBM.
3. A writing utensil for the student or computer to enter responses.
4. A writing utensil and clipboard for the teacher/examiner.
5. A stopwatch or countdown timer that displays seconds.
6. A quiet testing environment to work with students.
7. An equal-interval graph or a graphing program to plot the data.

M-CAP CBM Sheets

Similar to M-COMP CBM sheets, M-CAP CBM sheets are developed using a curricular sampling approach that results in SBMs. Specific item types should be aligned with the skills or content from the curriculum expected to be mastered by the end of the grade. The alternate forms should have different problems but be equivalent in complexity (i.e., at the same grade level). Therefore, each sheet is equivalent and represents the curriculum from the entire year (Fuchs & Fuchs, 1991).

One copy of each math sheet will be needed as well as an answer key for the teacher/ examiner that contains the correct answers and indicates the number of points associated with each problem. We recommend administering all universal screening assessments in one testing session to save setup time and for consistency in obtaining an accurate score, but it can occur across consecutive days if needed. If three samples of the same assessment are to be administered, then the median score is used for the final score and can also be placed as the first data point on the student's graph. After that, 20–30 different but equivalent sheets will be used to monitor student progress in math throughout the year.

M-CAP CBM can be administered individually or to a group. Two copies of the sheet will be needed. The student should have a pencil or pen and a copy of the M-CAP CBM sheet in front of him, and the teacher/examiner should have either a copy of the M-CAP CBM sheet in front of her on the computer screen or a paper copy to write on and a writing utensil, as well as a timer and the directions. See Figures 8.5 and 8.6 for examples of each type of sheet.

Directions and Scoring Procedures for M-CAP CBM

For your convenience, Appendix B includes a reproducible version of the directions and scoring rules for M-CAP CBM.

Directions for M-CAP CBM[3]

1. Place a copy of the student sheet in front of the students.
2. Say: *"The sheets on your desk have math problems on them. There are several types of math problems on the sheet. Look at each problem carefully before you answer it. When I say 'Please begin,' start answering the problems. Begin with the first problem and work in the order presented (point). If you cannot answer the problem, mark an 'X' through it and go to the next one. If you finish a page, turn the page and continue working until I say 'Thank you.' Are there any questions? Please begin."*
3. Once you say *"Please begin,"* start the countdown timer (*set for 6 minutes or the appropriate time limit*). At the end of the time limit, say: *"Thank you"* and have the students put their pencils down and stop working.

Scoring M-CAP CBM

Submit the results using the online system. Or:

1. Count the total number of problems attempted.
2. Count the total number of errors.

---

[3]Adapted with permission from Shinn (1989).

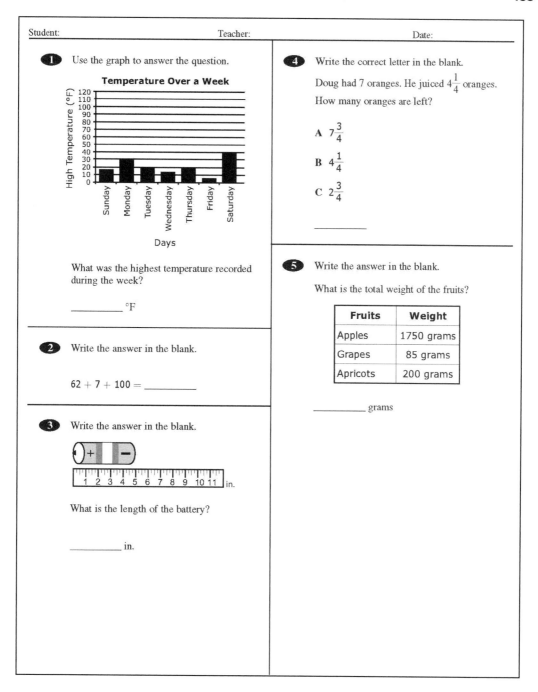

Student: Teacher: Date:

1   Use the graph to answer the question.

Temperature Over a Week

High Temperature (°F)

120
110
100
90
80
70
60
50
40
30
20
10
0

Sunday | Monday | Tuesday | Wednesday | Thursday | Friday | Saturday

Days

What was the highest temperature recorded during the week?

_____ °F

2   Write the answer in the blank.

62 + 7 + 100 = _____

3   Write the answer in the blank.

1 2 3 4 5 6 7 8 9 10 11   in.

What is the length of the battery?

_____ in.

4   Write the correct letter in the blank.

Doug had 7 oranges. He juiced $4\frac{1}{4}$ oranges. How many oranges are left?

A $7\frac{3}{4}$

B $4\frac{1}{4}$

C $2\frac{3}{4}$

_____

5   Write the answer in the blank.

What is the total weight of the fruits?

Fruits	Weight
Apples	1750 grams
Grapes	85 grams
Apricots	200 grams

_____ grams

FIGURE 8.5. Example of student M-CAP CBM sheet. Reprinted with permission from NCS Pearson.

Reminder: There is **no** partial credit when scoring. The answer must be correct **in its entirety** to obtain the correct score value. If any part of a multi-part question is incorrect, the score is zero.

Grade 4, Probe 1 Answer Key				Grade 4, Probe 2 Answer Key				Grade 4, Probe 3 Answer Key			
Item No.	Answer	Correct	Incorrect	Item No.	Answer	Correct	Incorrect	Item No.	Answer	Correct	Incorrect
1.	90	1	0	1.	70	1	0	1.	40	1	0
2.	427	1	0	2.	165	1	0	2.	169	1	0
3.	3	1	0	3.	8	1	0	3.	5	1	0
4.	C	2	0	4.	B	2	0	4.	C	2	0
5.	1,875	1	0	5.	1,895	1	0	5.	2035	1	0
6.	A	1	0	6.	A	1	0	6.	A	1	0
7.	38	2	0	7.	46	2	0	7.	50	2	0
8.	Indonesia	1	0	8.	Peru	1	0	8.	Canada	1	0
9.	9	3	0	9.	4	3	0	9.	9	3	0
10.	C	1	0	10.	B	1	0	10.	A	1	0
11.	1, 20	2	0	11.	1, 35	2	0	11.	1, 45	2	0
12.	7	1	0	12.	12	1	0	12.	16	1	0
13.	C	1	0	13.	B	1	0	13.	C	1	0
14.	5.60	2	0	14.	6	2	0	14.	6.30	2	0
15.	$\frac{6}{11}$	1	0	15.	$\frac{11}{11}$	1	0	15.	$\frac{6}{13}$	1	0
16.	B	1	0	16.	B	1	0	16.	A	1	0
17.	3	2	0	17.	6	2	0	17.	7	2	0
18.	4	1	0	18.	4	1	0	18.	9	1	0
19.	(2, 4)	2	0	19.	(2, 6)	2	0	19.	(10, 6)	2	0
20.	A	2	0	20.	C	2	0	20.	C	2	0
21.	91, 96	3	0	21.	44, 49	3	0	21.	77, 82	3	0
22.	B	1	0	22.	A	1	0	22.	A	1	0
23.	$\frac{1}{2}$ or 1:2 or 1 in 2	2	0	23.	$\frac{1}{4}$ or 1:4 or 1 in 4	2	0	23.	$\frac{1}{4}$ or 1:4 or 1 in 4	2	0
24.	A	1	0	24.	C	1	0	24.	B	1	0
25.	2	2	0	25.	2	2	0	25.	3	2	0
26.	A	2	0	26.	C	2	0	26.	B	2	0
27.	$\frac{1}{7}$	1	0	27.	$\frac{1}{11}$	1	0	27.	$\frac{1}{5}$	1	0
28.	B	3	0	28.	A	3	0	28.	A	3	0
29.	7	2	0	29.	4	2	0	29.	5	2	0
30.	C	3	0	30.	A	3	0	30.	C	3	0
Total				Total				Total			

FIGURE 8.6. Example of teacher/examiner M-CAP CBM sheet. Reprinted with permission from NCS Pearson.

3. Calculate rate: Total items attempted – total errors = total correct per time (6–10 minutes).
4. Calculate accuracy: Total correct ÷ total items attempted = percent correct.
5. Record the associated points for each correct problem for each student (as determined in the publisher's scoring manual).

When scoring M-CAP CBM, most publishers use a point system that weights correct problems based on the complexity of their solution and how much time might typically be used to solve them. Therefore, there are two ways of looking at results from M-CAP CBM, CP and points. Because there will be a pretty clear relation between the CP and points, we recommend using what the publisher recommends—most commonly points. Remember, when comparing your students' performance to the publisher's benchmarks or norms, it is crucial to use the same scoring metric, as those used to develop the benchmarks or norms.

SCORED AS CORRECT

• Answered correctly: Some publishers still use a production response (adhering to original CBM principles) such that the student needs to produce the response she thinks is correct by writing it in a blank. If this is the case, the student's response must be compared to that in the answer key. For the sake of simplicity and greater automation, some publishers are using a selected response format (i.e., multiple choice with three potential responses). This is a simplified format for computerized administration advances. Although within a framework of instructional hierarchy or Bloom's taxonomy this represents a different level of mastery of the task, preliminary research suggests similar technical adequacy. Given the savings in time for administration and scoring, this could increase utility of the measures. If the student has the correct answer, she is given credit for 1 CP, which will be converted to a predetermined number of points (generally 1–3) using a table in the scoring manual.
• Incomplete/crossed out: If a problem has been crossed out or started, but not completed, the student still receives appropriate credit. Correct work is correct work, even if the student did not finish the problem.
• Reversed/rotated: Reversed or rotated digits are scored as correct with the exception of 6's and 9's. With 6's and 9's, it is not possible to tell which one the student meant to write. No other digits can become others through rotation or reversal.

SCORED AS ERRORS

All errors are marked with a slash (/). See Figure 8.4 (panels D, E, and F) for three examples.

• Substitutions: When a student writes the wrong number.
• Omissions: Each number that is not recorded.

Special Administration and Scoring Considerations for M-CAP CBM

1. Correction procedure: If the student makes an error, he is not corrected. Particularly because M-CAP CBM can be administered to a group, error correction is not possible or appropriate.

2. Skip an entire page: If a student skips an entire page that page is not counted in the score. Because of the curriculum-sampling nature of M-CAP CBM, a student might not be able to complete the problems on that page. If this is the case, that is OK; however, it is important to check the student's work to ensure he is attempting problems that you know he has been exposed to in order to determine his skill with the task.

3. Discontinuation rule: Because some M-CAP CBM versions are using a multiple-choice format, one new concern is guessing. Similar to Maze, options for controlling for guessing could include using a discontinuation rule of two or three consecutive errors. However, the impact and utility of these strategies must be empirically tested before recommendations can be given. As usual, follow the publisher's guidelines, particularly when comparing student performance to publisher benchmarks or norms.

HOW OFTEN SHOULD MATH CBM BE ADMINISTERED?

In Chapter 2, we provide additional details on how often and when to administer CBM for the different purposes of universal screening and progress monitoring. Below we provide only an outline for these purposes. We suggest you refer to Chapter 2 for a more in-depth discussion on how often and when to give CBM for these different purposes.

Universal Screening

All students should be screened using grade level materials three times a year. This typically occurs in fall, winter, and spring. Universal screening data assist in answering some important questions, two of which are:

> "Is this student *at risk* for academic failure by the end of the year?"
> "Is our core instruction meeting the needs of most of our students?"

Progress Monitoring

Only those students who have been identified as *at risk*, meaning they did not score at or above the benchmark score on the universal screening assessment, should be progress monitored at least once a week on instructional level material and at least once per month on grade level materials if it is different from instructional level. An important aspect of progress monitoring is to do it often (i.e., weekly) and consistently (i.e., using CBM materials that are at the same difficulty level). Progress monitoring data assist in answering two very important questions:

"Is this student benefiting from the instruction she is receiving?"

"Is this intervention helping the majority of the students who have received it?"

HOW MUCH TIME DOES IT TAKE TO ADMINISTER AND SCORE MATH CBM?

The time needed to score each student sheet is the same for M-COMP CBM and M-CAP CBM. If you are giving a test to a class of 25 students or an individual student, the time limit for student performance of the task is the same (according to publisher recommendations). Given the time required to distribute the materials, read the directions, and have students hand in their work, we estimate this process, once the students are familiar with it, should take about 5 minutes in addition to the administration time limit.

Having a predetermined answer key is vital to accurate and efficient scoring. All publishers provide these. It will not be necessary to count the CD for each problem if they are all calculated correctly. If the student made some errors, we recommend counting the identified CD rather than subtracting the errors from the total potential CD. The most common scoring error that we see is a missing digit not being scored as an error. If counting CD, this doesn't affect the total; if subtracting errors from the total CD, it provides a higher score than earned. In the example below, the scorer correctly identified the digit written as incorrect but forgot to note that the correct answer (20) has 2 CD, meaning that the blank space to the left of the 8 is an incorrect digit. If counting CD, this has no effect on the total. If counting the number of errors and subtracting them from the total possible CD, it would lead to a total that is one greater than what the student actually earned. Multiple errors of this type would add up and introduce a systematic bias in one's scores.

$$
\begin{array}{r}
14 \\
+\ 6 \\
\hline
\cancel{8}
\end{array}
$$

0 CD-S
0 CD-A
0 CP
2 errors

As with most things, you will become more proficient with practice. In our experience it should take no longer than 1–2 minutes to score Math CBM for each student.

MATH CBM SCORES

There is currently no research on benchmarks for any of the M-COMP CBM or M-CAP curriculum-based measures (aimsweb publishes "default cut scores," but these are norms using the 45th and 15th percentile rather than empirically derived cut scores). If you remember from Chapter 2, we indicated that benchmarks are helpful because they are predictive of later student achievement. This allows teachers to determine who is on track and who needs additional assistance to be successful in math.

In the absence of empirically derived benchmarks, norms are the best currently available option. The norms are helpful because they provide a way of comparing a student's score to the performance of others in his grade or at his instructional level. The norms can then be used to determine how much growth we would expect a student to demonstrate to either maintain his level of relative performance or close the gap between his performance and his peers'. Table 8.1 provides information on norms for M-CAP CBM for grade 1 through grade 6.

HOW DO I USE THE INFORMATION TO WRITE MATH IEP GOALS AND OBJECTIVES?

Using the same format presented in Chapter 2, here are some examples of goals derived from Math CBM data. The principles are the same: time, learner, behavior (e.g., calculates, adds, subtracts), level (e.g., grade), content (e.g., math), material (Math CBM progress monitoring material), and criteria (will reflect the norms or benchmarks for that skill including time and accuracy).

Example of Goals
- Math goal
  - In 30 weeks, Larry will calculate addition and subtraction problems from second-grade mixed-operation M-COMP CBM progress monitoring material at 45 CD in 2 minutes with greater than 95% accuracy.

The same principles apply when writing objectives, but one should use a shorter time frame.

Example of Objective
- Objective goal
  - In 10 weeks, Larry will calculate addition and subtraction problems from second-grade mixed-operation M-COMP CBM progress-monitoring material at 25 CD in 2 minutes with greater than 95% accuracy.

SPECIAL CONSIDERATIONS THAT APPLY TO MATH CBM
Accuracy of Teacher/Examiner Copy

Because the teacher's/examiner's copy is invaluable and time saving, it is critically important that it be correct. This sounds like common sense, but it is very important to make sure that the answers to the problems and the number of CD or points assigned to them are all

TABLE 8.1. Norms for M-CAP CBM

Grade	Percentile	aimsweb (2015)		
		Fall (Points)	Winter (Points)	Spring (Points)
2	90%	17	31	36
	75%	11	24	30
	50%	**7**	**16**	**21**
	25%	4	11	14
	10%	2	6	9
3	90%	13	19	28
	75%	10	15	21
	50%	**7**	**11**	**15**
	25%	4	7	11
	10%	3	5	8
4	90%	21	27	33
	75%	16	21	24
	50%	**12**	**16**	**18**
	25%	9	12	13
	10%	6	9	9
5	90%	15	20	21
	75%	11	15	15
	50%	**8**	**11**	**11**
	25%	6	8	7
	10%	4	6	5
6	90%	24	31	35
	75%	18	24	27
	50%	**13**	**17**	**19**
	25%	9	12	13
	10%	6	9	9
7	90%	19	26	30
	75%	14	20	24
	50%	**10**	**15**	**18**
	25%	7	11	13
	10%	4	7	9
8	90%	19	23	26
	75%	14	17	20
	50%	**10**	**12**	**13**
	25%	6	7	9
	10%	4	4	5

correct—*even if you have gotten premade sheets*. One of us was using a set of premade sheets downloaded for free. One of the forms had been used about five or six times before a scoring error was noticed. The error reduced the CD for one problem by 2. This may not seem like much, but when comparing that sheet to others (such as during progress monitoring), it will systematically underestimate a student's performance.

Setting Up M-COMP CBM Sheets to Provide Potential Diagnostic Information

Unlike reading or writing, math is easier to separate into discrete skills. Therefore, when developing math CBM sheets, it is prudent to plan so that the results can be used in a diagnostic way. This is easier to accomplish for M-COMP CBM than for M-CAP CBM because the items are consistent in size and reading is not necessary. Take our example of aligning the math sheet with our curriculum. We were able to identify five skills that needed to be included. Our sheet was easily set up into five columns and five rows, giving us a total of 25

BOX 8.2. Websites for Creating Math CBM Sheets

AplusMath (*www.aplusmath.com*). Has premade single-operation sheets for computation, decimals, fractions, money, and algebra. Some also available as online sheets that are automatically scored. Also contains a worksheet generator to make mixed-operation sheets.

Intervention Central (*www.interventioncentral.org/teacher-resources/math-work-sheet-generator*). Generates single-operation or mixed-operation sheets. Allows detailed selection of problem types. Can be included in order selected or randomized. Also allows you to set number of rows and columns.

Math-Aids.Com (*www.math-aids.com*). Can generate single-operation or mixed-operation sheets. Also allows for many other math skills, including fractions, measurement, money, number lines, ratios, telling time, and word problems. Some customization is allowed. This is a free service, but it also offers a service for a fee that eliminates ads and provides faster downloads.

The Math Worksheet Site (*themathworksheetsite.com*). Can generate single-operation or mixed-operation sheets. Also allows for fractions, measurement, graphing, and telling time. Not much control in creating sheets. There is also a subscription-access-only area with many other types of sheets and skills available.

SuperKids (*superkids.com/aweb/tools/math*). Has generators for single-operation sheets and a mixed addition/subtraction version. No other mixed-operation capabilities. Also has generators for fractions, greater than/less than, rounding, averages, and telling time. Provides basic, advanced (includes negative numbers and decimals), and horizontal versions for computation skills.

Schoolhouse Technologies (*www.schoolhousetech.com*). Free resources include basic facts worksheet factory with addition, subtraction, multiplication, multiplication/division, and mixed options. Rather than creating sheets online, this is a program to download and run on your own computer. Pay version includes many more skills and options for customizing sheets.

problems. We then took all of those five skills and put them on a diagonal (see Figure 8.7). This way, as we score the sheet, we can look to see if there is a pattern of the student missing problems within a diagonal. If the student misses all of the problems in a diagonal, we should check to see if she has been taught that skill yet. If so, it might be one that she needs additional instruction on or practice with. We could also look to determine if the student has difficulty with the basic facts that support a certain skill or multiple skills. This is often the case when the student has difficulty doing multidigit problems that involve borrowing or carrying (although it might also be an issue of place value or the process of borrowing/carrying). Again, these patterns should not be considered reliable evidence of that student's deficit in the specific skills, but should be considered as hypotheses to test with more in-depth measures (such as a single-operation sheet) or evidence of skills that need to be taught or reviewed. (The adage we like to adhere to is "When in doubt, teach."). For additional information on how identify skills to be taught, please refer to *The ABCs of Curriculum-Based Evaluation* (Hosp et al., 2014).

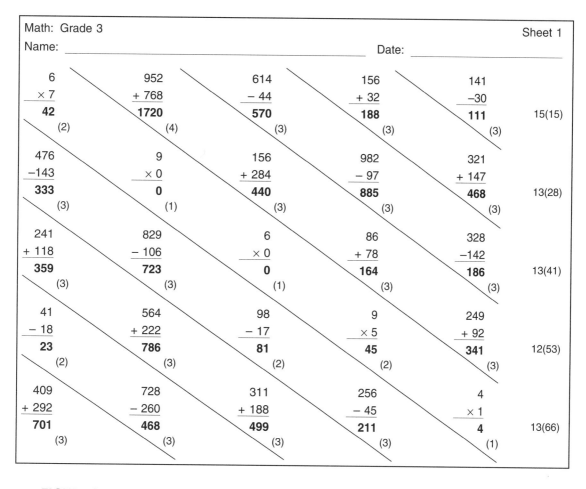

FIGURE 8.7. Example of a mixed-operation CBM sheet set up for diagnostic decision making.

Estimation

One of the concepts included in M-CAP CBM is estimation. This is an important math skill that is being explored as a useful criterion measure because it is thought to be a good indicator of number sense. Estimation sheets generally consist of 40 problems (both word and computation format) with three answers provided. One of the answers is close to the correct answer (how close it is varies) but not exact, and the other two are further away. Students are to identify which of the provided answers is closest to the correct answer. They have 3 minutes to complete as many of the problems as possible.

Algebra

In addition to estimation, algebra is a component of math that used to be thought of as an isolated content area (typically taught in high school) but is now recognized as a foundation of much of mathematics. Development work has yielded three types of Algebra CBM. Algebra Basic Skills (ABS) includes some of the foundational concepts and skills that serve as prerequisites to algebra (e.g., combining like terms, distributive property). Algebra Foundations (AF) includes the skills in the ABS measure and also algebra-specific skills such as coordinate graphs and data/function tables. These two measures are composed of constructed response items, and the student is given 5 minutes to complete as many as she can. Algebra Content Analysis (ACA) includes more advanced topics in algebra such as determining the slope of a line given two points and solving systems of equations in two variables. It is composed of multiple-choice items with partial credit awarded for work that is shown. Students are given 7 minutes to work on this measure.

FREQUENTLY ASKED QUESTIONS ABOUT MATH CBM

1. *Do teachers generally administer Math CBM sheets one on one with each student or to a group?* It depends on the teacher and the purpose. When universally screening a whole class, it makes more sense to administer to the entire group. When doing weekly progress monitoring, you might do it individually or with a small group of two to three students.

2. *My student has improved her math performance as I have monitored her progress, but she is not receiving any instruction in math. Could assessing using CBM alone be making a difference?* The extra 2–10 minutes of "practice" that she is getting per week is probably not enough to show improvement. She may be practicing elsewhere or receiving additional instruction.

3. *I only have 20 Math CBM sheets, but I need to progress monitor for 35 weeks. Is it OK to use the same sheets again?* Yes. Once you have used all 20, start using them again. The student probably doesn't remember specific items she did 20 weeks ago. This also means that you should not use the math sheets as homework or additional practice if you want to use them again.

4. *Should I tell my students that they get credit for each part of the computation problems rather than just correct/incorrect for the problem?* No, because it's the answer that is the most important part. If a student is concentrating on the intermediate stages even though she can calculate a complex problem in her head, she may show work she doesn't need to. This would slow her down by adding unnecessary steps. You want to get the most authentic measure of the student's performance.

5. *Because Math CBM measures automaticity, skipping time-consuming problems might be a calculated choice so that the student can move on to problems that can be solved more quickly. Does not answering specific questions really indicate a gap in skills or could it be a logical strategy?* More complex problems have more CD or points associated with them, so it's a flawed strategy anyway. If a student is skipping certain types of problems, you should administer a single-operation sheet to determine if she can't or won't do that type of problem. Sometimes the solution is as simple as asking the student, "Why did you skip these problems?" If her answer is "So I could finish more of the easier ones," you should remind her to attempt every problem and have her do another sheet.

6. *Can I use benchmark scores on Math CBM to put students in instructional groups?* Yes, if you have students with similar instructional needs. These groups should be flexible and students should be evaluated and regrouped every 6–8 weeks.

7. *Not everyone in my class is on the same instructional level. Should I still give them all the same Math CBM sheets?* All students should be screened/benchmarked on their grade level, but they should be progress monitored on their instructional level, especially if they are receiving instruction on that level. The best way to handle this is to give both the grade-level and the instructional-level math sheets each week so that you have an indication of how students are doing given the instruction they are receiving (instructional level) and how well it is transferring to more complex problems (grade level).

8. *What should I do with the scored sheets?* This information can be kept in a portfolio along with the graphed data to demonstrate progress over the year.

RESOURCES AND/OR FURTHER READING

AplusMath (*www.aplusmath.com*). Has premade single-skill sheets for computation, decimals, fractions, money, and algebra. Some are available as online sheets that are automatically scored. Also contains a worksheet generator to make mixed-math sheets.

Calhoon, M. (2008). Curriculum-based measurement for mathematics at the high school level: What we do not know . . . what we need to know. *Assessment for Effective Intervention, 33*, 234–239.

Christ, T., Scullin, S., Tolbize, A., & Jiban, C. (2008). Implications of recent research: Curriculum-based measurement of math computation. *Assessment for Effective Intervention, 33*, 198–205.

Foegen, A. (2008). Progress monitoring in middle school mathematics: Options and issues. *Remedial and Special Education, 29*, 195–207.

Foegen, A., Jiban, C., & Deno, S. (2007). Progress monitoring measures in mathematics: A review of the literature. *Journal of Special Education, 41*, 121–139.

Foegen, A., & Morrison, C. (2010). Putting algebra progress monitoring into practice: Insights from the field. *Intervention in School and Clinic, 46*, 95–103.

Fuchs, L. S., Fuchs, D., Hamlett, C. L., & Stecker, P. M. (1990). The role of skills analysis in curriculum-based measurement in math. *School Psychology Review, 19*, 6–22.

Fuchs, L. S., Fuchs, D., Hamlett, C. L., Thompson, A., Roberts, P. H., Kubek, P., et al. (1994). Technical features of a mathematics concepts and applications curriculum-based measurement system. *Diagnostique, 19*(4), 23–49.

Fuchs, L. S., Fuchs, D., & Zumeta, R. (2008). A curricular-sampling approach to progress monitoring: Mathematics concepts and applications. *Assessment for Effective Intervention, 33*, 225–233.

Intervention Central (*www.interventioncentral.org/teacher-resources/math-work-sheet-generator*). Generates single-skill or mixed-math sheets. Allows detailed selection of problem types. Can be included in order selected or randomized. Also allows you to set number of rows and columns.

Math-Aids.Com (*www.math-aids.com*). Can generate single-skill or mixed-math sheets. Also allows for many other math skills, including fractions, measurement, money, number lines, ratios, telling time, and word problems. Some customization is allowed. This is a free service, but it also offers a service for a fee that eliminates ads and provides faster downloads.

The Math Worksheet Site (*themathworksheetsite.com*). Can generate single-skill or mixed-math sheets. Also allows for fractions, measurement, graphing, and telling time. Not much control in creating sheets. There is also a subscription-access-only area with many other types of sheets and skills available.

Schoolhouse Technologies (*www.schoolhousetech.com*). Free resources include basic facts worksheet factory with addition, subtraction, multiplication, multiplication/division, and mixed options. Rather than creating sheets online, this is a program to download and run on your own computer. Pay version includes many more skills and options for customizing sheets.

SuperKids (*superkids.com/aweb/tools/math*). Has generators for single-skill sheets and a mixed addition/subtraction version. No other mixed-math capabilities. Also has generators for fractions, greater than/less than, rounding, averages, and telling time. Provides basic, advanced (includes negative numbers and decimals), and horizontal versions for computation skills.

Thurber, R. S., Shinn, M. R., & Smolkowski, K. (2002). What is measured in mathematics tests? Construct validity of curriculum-based mathematics measures. *School Psychology Review, 31*, 498–513.

VanDerHeyden, A. M., & Burns, M. K. (2005). Using curriculum-based assessment and curriculum-based measurement to guide elementary mathematics instruction: Effect on individual and group accountability scores. *Assessment for Effective Intervention, 30*, 15–31.

CHAPTER 9

How to Conduct Content-Area CBM

WHY SHOULD I CONDUCT CONTENT-AREA CBM?

Because of the emphasis on basic skills and its use with students who are struggling or receiving special education services, CBM has predominantly focused on the elementary grades and the core subjects of reading, math, writing, and spelling. But as CBM's utility has expanded to middle and high school, an additional emphasis on content-area performance has increased. As discussed in Chapter 8, a suite of curriculum-based measures for algebra have been developed: Algebra Basic Skills (ABS), Algebra Foundations (AF), and Algebra Content Analysis (ACA). For other content areas, CBM approaches have been developed that can be used with history and science but are not specific to either of these or other content areas.

With the Common Core State Standards and Next Generation Science Standards, foundational skills such as reading and math are expected to be infused into content-area instruction. This puts an additional assessment demand on content-area teachers, particularly in the secondary grades. It is especially important for students who struggle with reading because they will need to read and comprehend in order to access the content-area material. Use of various measures to access both reading and content knowledge is promising for universal screening and progress monitoring in the secondary grades.

OPR AND MAZE CBM

The most common approaches to Content-Area CBM have been to take informational text from a content area (e.g., history or science textbooks) and format them as OPR CBM or Maze CBM passages. The requirements for materials, directions, and scoring with this approach are all consistent with those presented in Chapter 4. There is some disagreement about the utility of this approach, however, because of concerns with alignment. For OPR CBM, predictive utility often declines beginning in grade 4 due to a leveling off of how automatically individuals can read text. More research is needed in this area before recommendations for or against OPR CBM for content areas can be made.

The declining predictive utility of OPR CBM beyond grade 4 is one reason Maze is considered a preferable option. There is some disagreement about whether Maze is a direct measure of comprehension or of silent reading. However, like OPR CBM, it is a viable indicator of comprehension or overall reading performance. More research is needed to determine how well a content-area Maze passage predicts comprehension within the content area, but one advantage Maze CBM might have over OPR CBM is that the task of restoring the appropriate words in the blanks may tap into the use of academic vocabulary. This is the foundation of another approach to Content-Area CBM, Vocabulary Matching CBM.

VOCABULARY MATCHING CBM

Vocabulary Matching CBM uses important terms and definitions within a content area as an indicator of performance within the content. Automaticity with academic vocabulary is considered a foundational skill within content areas in the same way that decoding and computation are foundational skills for reading and math, respectively. When a student can quickly and accurately determine what key vocabulary terms mean, she can dedicate more attention and effort to reasoning and application.

Materials Needed to Conduct Vocabulary Matching CBM

1. Different but equivalent stimuli sheets (student and teacher/examiner copies).
2. Directions for administering and scoring Vocabulary Matching CBM.
3. A writing utensil for the student.
4. A writing utensil and clipboard.
5. A stopwatch or countdown timer that displays seconds.
6. A quiet testing environment to work with students.
7. An equal-interval graph or a graphing program to plot the data.

Vocabulary Matching CBM Sheets

Vocabulary Matching CBM sheets include vocabulary terms and their definitions that are drawn directly from the materials used for instruction in the content areas. These can include textbooks and other reading materials, teacher notes and plans, state standards (or in the case of science, the Next Generation Science Standards), and/or district guidelines. These materials are presented in a matching format that includes terms and definitions that the student must match.

Each sheet typically includes 20 vocabulary terms in a column on the left side of the page with their associated definitions along with two distractor definitions in a column on the right. The presentation order of the 22 definitions should be random. Each definition should have a short blank next to its item number for the student to record the letter of the corresponding definition (see Figure 9.1).

Science Vocabulary Matching

Name: _____   Date: _____

_____ Electromagnet

_____ Compound

_____ Kelvin

_____ Diffraction

_____ Lithosphere

a. The process by which a green plant turns water and carbon dioxide into food when the plant is exposed to light.

b. The cultivation of aquatic organisms (generally fish or shellfish), especially for food.

c. A substance formed by the chemical union of two or more ingredients in specific proportion.

d. A tide of minimum range occurring at the first and third quarters of the moon.

FIGURE 9.1. Example of student Vocabulary Matching CBM sheet.

We recommend administering all universal screening assessments in one testing session to save setup time and for consistency in obtaining an accurate score, but it can occur across consecutive days if needed. If three samples of the same assessment are to be administered, then the median score is used for the final score and can also be placed as the first data point on the student's graph. After that, 20–30 different but equivalent sheets will be used to monitor student progress in reading throughout the year.

Vocabulary Matching CBM can be administered individually or to a group. Two copies of the sheet will be needed. The student should have a copy of the Vocabulary Matching CBM sheet in front of him, and the teacher/examiner should have either a copy of the Vocabulary Matching CBM sheet in front of her on the computer screen or a paper copy to write on and a writing utensil, as well as a timer, and the directions. See Figures 9.1 and 9.2 for examples of each type of sheet.

Science Vocabulary Matching
Teacher/Examiner Copy

Q	Electromagnet
C	Compound
M	Kelvin
F	Diffraction
V	Lithosphere
B	Aquaculture
D	Neap tide
A	Photosynthesis

FIGURE 9.2. Example of teacher/examiner Vocabulary Matching CBM sheet.

Directions and Scoring Procedures for Vocabulary Matching CBM

For your convenience, Appendix B includes a reproducible version of the directions and scoring rules for Vocabulary Matching CBM.

Directions for Vocabulary Matching CBM

1. Place the student copy in front of the student(s).
2. Say: *"Look at the paper in front of you. There are vocabulary words on the left* (point to the column of vocabulary words) *and definitions for those words are on the right* (point to the column of definitions). *The definitions are in a mixed-up order, but every vocabulary word has its appropriate definition in the right column."*
3. Say: *"When I say begin, I want you to write the letter of the definition in the blank in front of the appropriate vocabulary word* (demonstrate by pointing). *Try each one. If you come to one that you don't know, you can come back to it. Are there any questions? Begin."* (Trigger timer for 5 minutes.)
4. If the student comes to the end of the page, make sure he continues working until the time is up.
5. At the end of 5 minutes, say *"Stop."*

Scoring Vocabulary Matching CBM

1. Count the total number of correct matches.

SCORED AS CORRECT

- Letter representing the correct definition for the vocabulary term.

SCORED AS ERRORS

- Letter representing an incorrect definition for the vocabulary term.
- Letter representing a distractor definition.

Special Administration and Scoring Considerations for Vocabulary Matching CBM

1. Correction procedure: If the student makes an error, she is *not* corrected.
2. Skip an entire row/line: If the student skips an entire row that row is not included in the scoring. If the student is skipping items, the examiner should say *"Make sure you try all the items."* If the student still does not attempt an item, or time runs out, do not count any uncompleted items.
3. Discontinuation Rule: There is no discontinuation rule for Vocabulary Matching CBM.

4. Finish before time limit: If the student finishes responding before 5 minutes, his rate score should be prorated. The formula for prorating is:

$$\frac{\text{Total number of correct definitions}}{\text{Number of seconds it took to finish}} \times 300 = \text{Estimated number of correct definitions}$$

Example: The student finished the sheet in 4½ minutes (270 seconds) and correctly identified 18 definitions.

$$\frac{18}{270} \times 300 = 20$$

We estimate that the student would have completed approximately 20 vocabulary matching items in 5 minutes had we provided more problems and timed her for the full 5 minutes.

HOW OFTEN
SHOULD CONTENT-AREA CBM BE ADMINISTERED?

In Chapter 2, we provide additional details on how often and when to administer CBM for the different purposes of universal screening and progress monitoring. Below we provide only an outline for these purposes. We suggest you refer to Chapter 2 for a more in-depth discussion on how often and when to give CBM for these different purposes.

Universal Screening

All students in a classroom or grade level should be screened once per quarter (three to four times per school year); typically conducted in the fall, winter, and spring. Universal screening data assist in answering some important questions, two of which are:

"Is this student *at risk* for academic failure by the end of the year?"
"Is our core instruction meeting the needs of most of our students?"

Progress Monitoring

Only those students who have been identified as *at risk*, meaning they did not score at or above the benchmark score on the universal screening assessment, should be progress monitored at least once a week on instructional level material and at least once per month on grade level materials if it is different from instructional level. An important aspect of progress monitoring is to do it often (i.e., weekly) and consistently (i.e., using CBM materials that are at the same difficulty level). Progress monitoring data assist in answering two very important questions:

"Is this student benefiting from the instruction he or she is receiving?"

"Is this intervention helping the majority of the students who have received it?"

HOW MUCH TIME DOES IT TAKE TO ADMINISTER AND SCORE CONTENT-AREA CBM?

When using OPR CBM or Maze CBM as a Content-Area CBM, the administration and scoring demands are the same as for Reading CBM. For Vocabulary Matching CBM, whether administering to an individual or a group, the time is similar. Once the students have the materials in front of them, the directions take less than 1 minute and administration 5 minutes. As indicated in Chapter 2, you will also need to factor in time for the student to move to where the teacher/examiner is or to distribute the materials. Having everything printed out and ready to go with the students' names already indicated on the appropriate forms (either handwritten or using printed labels) saves a lot of time. Scoring takes less than 1 minute per form as there are only a maximum of 20 items to check.

CONTENT-AREA CBM SCORES

Benchmarks for Content-Area CBM

There is currently no research on benchmarks that are specific to any content-area measures. If you remember from Chapter 2, we indicated that benchmarks are helpful because they are predictive of later student achievement. This allows teachers to determine who is on track and who needs additional assistance to be successful in the content area. Because OPR CBM and Maze CBM use procedures from Reading CBM, it could be possible to use benchmarks for those measures. However, many Reading CBM passages are focused on literary (i.e., narrative) rather than informational (i.e., expository). Given the different nature of reading different types of text, there is some emerging evidence that use of benchmarks developed for one suite of curriculum-based measures should not be used with those from another suite.

Norms for Content-Area CBM

In the absence of empirically derived benchmarks, norms for Content-Area CBM are an alternative. The norms are helpful because they provide a way of comparing a student's score to the performance of others in her grade or at her instructional level. The norms can then be used to determine how much growth we would expect a student to make to either maintain her level of relative performance or close the gap between her performance and her peers'. Similar to benchmarks, norms developed for one set of materials or CBM suite should not be used with different materials. There are currently no national norms available for Content-Area CBM, leaving development of local norms as the only available option.

HOW DO I USE THE INFORMATION TO WRITE CONTENT-AREA IEP GOALS AND OBJECTIVES?

Using the same format presented in Chapter 2, here are some examples of using Content-Area CBM data to write goals and objectives. The principles are the same: time, learner, behavior (e.g., identifies, counts), level (e.g., grade), content (e.g., science), material (Content-Area CBM progress monitoring material), and criteria (will reflect the norms or benchmarks for that skill including time and accuracy).

Example of Goal

- Science Vocabulary Matching goal
  - In 30 weeks, Sierra will match science terms with their definition on a Vocabulary Matching CBM sheet at 15 matches in 5 minutes with greater than 95% accuracy.

The same principles apply when writing objectives, but one should use a shorter time frame.

Example of Objective

- Science Vocabulary Matching goal
  - In 10 weeks, Sierra will match science terms with their definition on a Vocabulary Matching CBM sheet at 5 matches in 5 minutes with greater than 95% accuracy.

SPECIAL CONSIDERATIONS THAT APPLY TO CONTENT-AREA CBM

Because the teacher's/examiner's copy is invaluable and time saving, it is critically important that it be correct. This sounds like common sense, but it is very important to make sure that the answers to the problems are all correct. This is particularly important if you have developed your own content-area Maze passages or vocabulary matching probes.

FREQUENTLY ASKED QUESTIONS ABOUT CONTENT-AREA CBM

1. ***Do teachers generally administer Content-Area CBM sheets one on one with each student or to a group?*** Most content-area curriculum-based measures can be administered to a group since they allow for a written response. The exception would be OPR CBM, which requires a verbal response and thus must be administered individually. When universally screening a whole class, it might make sense to administer to the entire group. When doing weekly progress monitoring, we recommend individual administration.

2. ***My student has improved her performance as I have monitored her progress, but she is not receiving any instruction in the content area. Could assessing using CBM alone***

be making a difference? The extra 1–5 minutes of "practice" that she is getting per week is probably not enough to show improvement. She may be practicing elsewhere or receiving additional instruction.

3. *I only have 20 Content-Area CBM sheets, but I need to progress monitor for 35 weeks. Is it OK to use the same sheets again?* Yes, provided the 20 forms sample content from across the instructional period (i.e., grade). Provided the content in each form is representative of the end-of-grade content to be learned, rather than each form sampling a specific unit or topic (in a mastery measurement format), you will get a consistent assessment of the student's performance and progress. Once you have used all 20, start using them again. The student probably doesn't remember specific items she did 20 weeks ago. This also means that you should not use the sheets as homework or additional practice.

4. *Because there are no benchmark scores on content-area curriculum-based measures, can I use norms to put students in instructional groups?* Yes, if you have students with similar instructional needs. These groups should be flexible and students should be evaluated and regrouped every 6–8 weeks.

5. *Not everyone in my class is on the same instructional level. Should I still give them all the same Content-Area CBM sheets?* Unlike foundational skills and content from the elementary grades, content-area standards are even more grade-specific. In general, all students you work with are expected to learn grade-level content. They will likely require different instruction and degrees of practice and scaffolding, but the standards are the same. However, if you are working with a student with a significant disability who is working toward alternate standards, it is important to use materials that are relevant for the curriculum for that student. It would also be helpful to give both the grade-level and the instructional-level measures each week so that you have an indication of how students are doing given the instruction they are receiving (instructional level) and how well it is transferring to grade-level content.

6. *What should I do with the scored sheets?* This information can be kept in a portfolio along with the graphed data to demonstrate progress over the year.

RESOURCES AND/OR FURTHER READING

Chung, S., & Espin, C. A. (2013). CBM progress monitoring in foreign-language learning for secondary-school students: Technical adequacy of different measures and scoring procedures. *Assessment for Effective Intervention, 38,* 236–248.

Espin, C. A., Busch, T., Lembke, E. S., Hampton, D., Seo, K., & Zukowski, B. A. (2013). Curriculum-based measurement in science learning: Vocabulary-matching as an indicator of performance and progress. *Assessment for Effective Intervention, 38,* 203–213.

Espin, C. A., Shin, J., & Busch, T. (2005). Curriculum-based measurement in the content areas: Vocabulary matching as an indicator of progress in social studies learning. *Journal of Learning Disabilities, 29,* 570–581.

Mooney, P., McCarter, K., Schraven, J., & Haydel, B. (2010). The relationship between content area general outcome measurement and statewide testing in sixth-grade world history. *Assessment for Effective Intervention, 35,* 148–158.

Twyman, T., & Tindal, G. (2007). Extending curriculum-based measurement into middle/secondary schools: The technical adequacy of the concept maze. *Journal of Applied School Psychology, 24,* 49–67.

CHAPTER 10

Charting and Graphing Data to Help Make Decisions

Getting assessment data into a form that is easy to interpret and use is one of the most important things to consider. If the data we collect are not easy to use, we will be less likely to use them, and if we do not use them, why bother collecting them? One of the main benefits of CBM is that the data are displayed in graphs and charts (which are a lot easier to read and interpret than a page full of numbers). Different types of graphs can be used to examine the data in different ways. For example, line graphs are an excellent way to represent an individual's performance over time. They can also be used to show a group's performance over time. However, for universal screening decisions (which are more static than progress decisions) box plots, histograms, and pie charts are more common. This chapter demonstrates some types of graphs that are commonly used to display CBM data and some decision rules for using them.

COMMON GRAPHS FOR DISPLAYING CBM DATA

Line Graphs

The original type of graph used with CBM is a typical line graph like the one in Figure 10.1. We have included a blank copy to reproduce/download in Appendix B. The vertical axis of the graph (marked as "Words Read Correctly"—the ordinate in a plane Cartesian coordinate system, for you math-o-philes) indicates the number correct on a CBM probe. The actual metric will be different for different content areas (e.g., WRC is the OPR metric for Reading CBM). The increments should be sized so that student growth can be accurately observed. Increments that are too large may understate the student's growth, and increments that are too small may overstate it. The horizontal axis (marked as "# of weeks"—the abscissa) is used to indicate the number of weeks the student will be monitored, allowing for data to be entered one to two times per week.

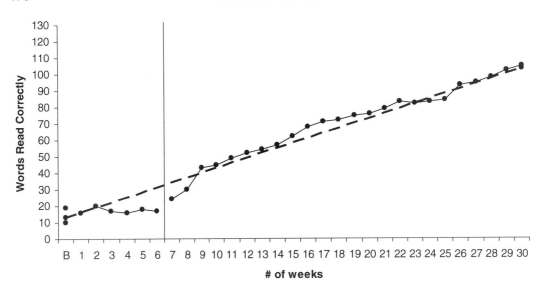

FIGURE 10.1. Example of CBM line graph.

Because the chart has both a time axis (number of weeks) and a skill axis (WRC), it allows us to record changes in student learning over time. Learning (or a lack of it) is what we begin to see as we collect a series of data points. This is significant because it means that by charting CBM results we get two kinds of data: data on student level of performance, and data on student rate of progress. Performance scores tell us how well a student can do that task. Progress scores tell us how quickly she is learning how to perform it.

For each content area, a separate graph using the same scale should be used for each student. Figure 10.2 illustrates why. The two graphs in Figure 10.2 use the same student data. Because the vertical axis of the graph on the right only goes from 0 to 30, the student

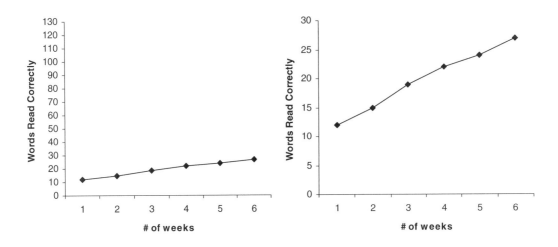

FIGURE 10.2. Student data plotted on graphs with different vertical axes.

appears to be making good progress (i.e., the trend of his progress is quite steep). When we examine his progress on the graph with the vertical axis that goes from 0 to 130, it doesn't look so good. In actuality, his progress is below his peers', and the decision should be that he is *not* making adequate progress.

Box Plots

Box plots (also called boxplots or box-and-whisker plots) are a way of illustrating the performance of a group. Figure 10.3 shows why they are called box plots. The middle of the box is the median score of the group (i.e., the score at the 50th percentile), while the top and bottom represent the 75th and 25th percentiles, respectively. This makes the three horizontal lines forming the rectangular box represent the 1st, 2nd, and 3rd quartiles (the statistical points that divide a group into four equal parts). This means that, by definition, the performance of half of the students in the group falls within the box.

The vertical lines sticking out of the top and bottom (the whiskers) extend the range to show values closer to the maximum and minimum. There is less of a convention on how far these should extend. Using the 10th and 90th percentile is one option (although this leaves 20 percent of the students outside the graphic), but the 2nd and 98th are also fairly common. This is probably because they represent two standard deviation units away from the mean in each direction. Less common is using the minimum and maximum scores. One reason this is less common is that it makes it difficult to determine how many students fell at the extremes because they are included in the whiskers. When not using the minimum and maximum values for the whiskers, any student whose performance falls outside the range of the whiskers is represented by an X or a dot.

Box plots can be particularly useful for universal screening data because they allow one to compare the performance of an entire group to the cut score or benchmark.

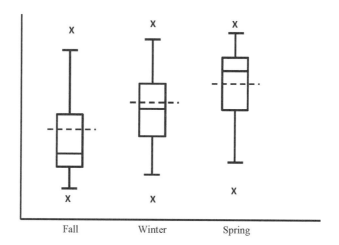

FIGURE 10.3. Example of CBM box plots.

Bar Charts

Bar charts are a common way of illustrating individual performance aggregated to a group level. Although many CBM suites and data management tools do not incorporate bar charts, they are incredibly helpful for educators who need to make decisions about groups and subgroups of students.

In a bar chart, each student is represented by a bar (seems clear why it's called a bar chart, doesn't it?). The bars can be sorted many different ways, but we recommend lowest score to highest. See Figure 10.4 for an example. The vertical axis should be whatever the CBM metric used is—in this case WRC. If we insert a horizontal line where the benchmark or cut score for proficiency is, then we have a visual representation of the proportion of students below that cut score as well as how far below they are. We also get to see how many students and which ones are above the cut score for proficiency. For a more detailed discussion of using bar charts to make decisions about groups and subgroups of students, we refer you to *The ABCs of Curriculum-Based Evaluation* (Hosp et al., 2014).

HOW TO CHART CBM DATA FOR PROGRESS MONITORING

Progress monitoring data should always include two pieces of information: first, the number correct, usually rate based, and second, the accuracy score (or number of errors). Proficiency in any skill includes an appropriate correct response rate and an appropriate level of accuracy. We can't think of *any* skill, including cooking, sports, music, or academics, where mastery of the skill does not include rate and accuracy. For example, see if you think these second-grade students have the same level of skills. Student A completes an OPR with 100 WRC at 95% accuracy; Student B completes an OPR with 100 WRC at 70% accuracy. Or Student A completes an OPR with 100 WRC at 95% accuracy and Student B completes an OPR with 80 WRC at 95% accuracy. Both rate and accuracy tell you how the student is

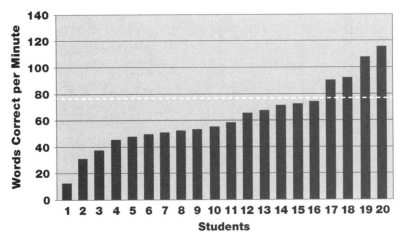

Ms. Allen's 3rd Grade Winter Benchmark Performance

FIGURE 10.4. Example of CBM bar chart.

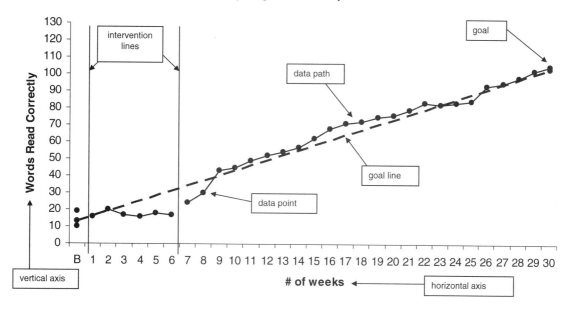

FIGURE 10.5. Sample CBM graph with each part labeled.

doing. Two chefs bake bread every day. Baker A always has his bread ready by 8 A.M. (rate) without any burnt loafs (accuracy). Baker B only has his bread ready half of the time by 8 A.M. (rate) without any burnt loafs (accuracy). Who is the better baker? I guess it depends if you like bread or not.

Figure 10.5 is an example of a CBM graph with each part of the graph labeled. The first thing we enter on the graph is the student's baseline data (the first column on the left side of the graph—marked with a B). This lets us know where the student is starting with his performance. To find the student's baseline, we administer three separate passages, lists, story starters, or sheets. Plot all three on the first vertical line. The one in the middle is the baseline score (if two scores are the same, that score is the baseline). Figure 10.5 shows that the three scores the student earned are 10, 13, and 19 along with the error scores (1, 0, 2) associated with each of his rate scores. His baseline score is therefore 13—the point from which we will start as well as 1 for errors.

HOW TO SET AND GRAPH GOALS
FOR PROGRESS MONITORING

Now that we have plotted the student's baseline data, we need to set a goal. There are three methods for setting goals: end-of-year benchmarks, norms (national or local), and intraindividual framework. Which method to use depends on the availability of information (Are there national norms?), the student's performance level (typically performing or at risk), and the comparison you want to make (to a performance criterion or a representative peer group). Below we provide a description for each, how to apply it, and what population you would want to use it with.

End-of-Year Benchmarks

The use of performance standards (i.e., benchmarks) is the preferred method of determining goals for those students who are behind. Benchmarks are cut scores that have been determined to reliably predict proficient performance on an external test in an area. The most common type of test to predict is currently state-mandated accountability tests that are used to determine whether or not a student has reached a predetermined level of proficiency or mastery as determined by the state. There are different methods of determining these cut scores for performance on the curriculum-based measures, but typically they determine the score at which a student has an 85% (or greater) probability of scoring above the criterion for proficiency on the outcome test.

Table 4.1 in Chapter 4 shows benchmarks for grades 1 through 6 for OPR CBM. At the end of the year, we want every student to be performing at or above the benchmark. For example, for a student in third grade, we would set our end-of-year goal at 100 WRC with at least 95% accuracy. This is the lowest score we would accept that would indicate a student is *not* at risk for future academic failure. Even if the students were not performing at an acceptable level at the beginning of the year (when we screened the class), as long as they make progress that will take them to mastery by the end of the year, we can feel confident that they will be performing proficiently and will not be at risk for difficulty in reading.

Benchmarks are generally the best method for setting goals because when they are well developed, they provide a consistent point for determining how likely it is that a student will meet proficiency requirements on a criterion measure (which should be linked to standards and/or other high-stakes decisions). There has been a huge increase in this type of psychometric work on different suites of curriculum-based measures, and it has become typical practice for anyone developing CBM materials.

Benchmarks are especially helpful for setting goals for those students who are behind. It allows the teacher to monitor weekly to determine if the student is "on track" to be successful by the end of the school year. For those students who are performing at or above the benchmark, you may not want to set their goal to the end-of-year benchmark as this may underestimate their performance. While these students are not typically progress monitored, if they were progress monitored it would be more appropriate to use an intraindividual process to calculate their end-of-year goal.

Norms

When benchmarks are not available, national norms can serve as a standard that can generalize to a broader population. Some effort has been made to identify national norms for CBM in most content areas, but less than that made to develop empirically derived benchmarks.

CBM has been used for more than 30 years, which has allowed for many researchers and publishers to collect large samples of scores that are representative of the U.S. school population. There are also CBM data sets representing only those who are using that particular CBM product, which tend to cover regional areas. Interestingly, the results from nationally represented and regionally represented CBM data sets appear to be remarkably similar. This type of CBM normative data allows you to set goals similar as you would using end-of-year benchmarks. The difference is that these are based on typical performance of same-grade peers rather than a criterion for proficiency that predicts performance on outcome measures (which is what benchmarks do). One finds the grade level the student is in, identifies the level of performance for the 50th percentile in the spring, and uses that as the end-of-year goal.

If national norms are not available, then local norms can be collected, and you can use the same process of finding the grade level and identifying the 50th percentile in spring to determine your end-of-year goal. Although we do not recommend using local norms, if you are interested in this option, Shinn (1989) provides information on it.

We would be remiss if we did not mention that historically there has also been work done to collect norms regarding rate of growth or progress. This has been calculated as an average weekly gain or rate of improvement (ROI). The ROI is then used to calculate the end-of-year goal by multiplying the rate by the number of weeks left until the aim date (i.e., the date by which you expect the student to reach the goal) and adding that number to the baseline score. However, we need to share our reservations about using progress norms. First, progress norms reflect the quality of instruction—more intense instruction should lead to greater growth. One thing we don't know about national progress norms is how good or intense the instruction was that the students were receiving. Second, the students who are farthest behind need to have the steepest slopes (i.e., the greatest rates of progress) in order to catch up to the expected level of performance, and progress norms may not represent the rate of growth needed.

Intraindividual Framework

The intraindividual framework uses the student's current level of performance and rate of progress to set end-of-year goals for his performance. While this method can be used, we caution that it may underestimate a student's rate of learning and may never catch her up if she started out behind. (Because she wasn't performing as well as she needed to is why we were concerned in the first place, right?) If the instruction is good and the student responds positively to it, using benchmarks or norms will provide better goals since they represent scores that are predictive of future academic success (i.e., benchmarks) or an indication of how other students at that grade level perform (i.e., norms). In our opinion, the only time you would want to use a student's past performance as a goal for future performance is when his past performance is average or above average, which is not typically true for the students whom we progress monitor.

In order to use an intrindividual framework you will need to collect at least eight data points and then subtract the lowest score from the highest. For example, if we were progress monitoring a second-grade student using OPR passages, his first eight scores might be 12, 16, 15, 19, 16, 21, 26, and 24. We find the difference: $26 - 12 = 14$. Divide this difference by the number of weeks (i.e., the number of data points we have collected, eight): $14 \div 8 = 1.75$. This baseline rate of growth is multiplied by 1.5 in order to set a weekly progress goal: $1.75 \times 1.5 = 2.625$. This number is then multiplied by the number of weeks left until the end of the year (or the end of the planned intervention. 2.625×16 weeks $= 42$. This number is then added to the median score of the first eight data points we used to calculate the baseline growth rate (it is 17.5—halfway between 16 and 19): 42 + 17.5 = 59.5. This is our end-of-year performance goal for this student: 59.5 (using 60 WRC as the goal ensures he scored above the goal).

GRAPHING GOALS

Now that we have set the goal for our student, we need to graph that goal on her chart. Whichever method we used to set the goal, we should have a specific target to work toward and a number of weeks we expect it will take to get there. These are the only two numbers we need to graph the student's goal. We will also want to graph the errors or accuracy to ensure the student is hitting the goal of 95% accuracy or better. As stated earlier both rate and accuracy contribute to the success of students' skills and need to be included when determining student growth and proficiency toward end-of-year goals. We also need to make sure that the paper we are using has enough room horizontally for all the weeks of data we will be collecting and enough room vertically to record the student's performance all the way to the goal.

Look at Figure 10.5 again. We had already plotted our student's baseline data and found his baseline score to be 13. Say we are using the benchmark to determine his goal. Let's say the benchmark score for his grade on OPR CBM is 103. Since we are planning to monitor the progress of the student's performance for the entire school year, we have 30 weeks left. So 30 weeks times 3 WRC per week is 90 WRC. In 30 weeks, we expect the student to *increase* his WRC by 90. This means we add it to his baseline score (13). At week 30 on our chart, we draw an X or a target at 103 (90 + 13). We then connect the baseline score and the goal. This is the student's goal line (also sometimes referred to as an *aim line*).

Each time we administer at least one passage or probe to the student, we enter his rate and error score on the graph and connect it to the previous point associated with each score. These are data points and the data path. This allows each student to have his database, which is used to evaluate the effectiveness of the instruction he is receiving.

HOW OFTEN SHOULD DATA BE COLLECTED?

How frequently to collect data and graph them depends on three things. First, it depends on our purpose—is it to screen or progress monitor? If we are assessing and graphing to screen all students' performance, we typically use curriculum-based measures three times per year. This is the "checking vital signs" exercise designed to pick up potential problems but not to yield much information about how to correct those problems when they are found. This sort of testing doesn't need to be done often. If we are monitoring progress to guide instruction, we need frequent feedback, so more frequent measurement is needed.

Second, how frequently we collect and graph data depends on the importance of the task. High-importance tasks need frequent monitoring. If there are particular skills that are of great importance, we should monitor them more directly and frequently than we would monitor skills of lesser consequence (this is basically why we watch young children more closely when they are playing near a street than when they are playing in a fenced backyard). Reading and language are good examples of skill areas in which we can't afford to let students fall behind without noticing. Reading Roman numerals might not meet the same criterion.

Third, frequency of collecting and graphing data depends on the significance of a problem. As the student's difficulties increase and the need for effective instruction becomes more urgent, the need for more frequent monitoring is increased. The magnitude of a student's difficulty is illustrated by the size of the difference between her actual level of performance and the expected level of performance as well as her rate of progress. A student who is far behind but making rapid progress may actually be seen as having less of a problem than another student who is only moderately behind expectations but making little or no progress.

What this means is that while there are no hard-and-fast rules for the frequency of progress monitoring. It should be increased when the content is important and the student is at risk for future academic problems. Most people recommend universally screening three or four times per year on curriculum-based measures. Progress monitoring should be done at least once per week for the students receiving Tier 2 or Tier 3 intervention. For students who are performing and progressing well, the universal screening measures may be enough to monitor their progress.

Progress monitoring using curriculum-based measures has traditionally consisted of data collection once or twice per week, particularly for those students who are significantly behind their grade-level standards. In an attempt to provide more stability of scores and therefore a clearer slope of student growth, some researchers are advocating for collecting data every other week (or even less frequently), but using two probes and calculating the mean or three probes and using the median. Research is still developing about the impact these approaches have on teachers' decision making and its resultant impact on student learning. Psychometrically it may provide a more stable slope, but the consequences of this have yet to be determined.

DECISION RULES TO HELP EDUCATORS USE THE DATA TO INFORM INSTRUCTION

Notice that in Figure 10.5 there are also vertical lines that separate sections of the data. These are called *intervention lines*. Where an intervention line falls, the data points on either side are not connected by a data path. This is to help us remember that something changed at that point and to group the data points more easily. Each intervention line shows us the point at which a decision about the student's progress was made.

There are two methods of making decisions about whether the student's response to instruction is appropriate or not (i.e., if the student's progress is adequate for him to meet his goal within the expected time period). The first is data point analysis and the second is trend line analysis. With either method, the goal line is used as a reference point.

With data point analysis, the data points on the graph for each week are examined. After collecting an initial six to eight data points, any time four *consecutive* scores fall below the goal line, a decision needs to be made. This decision is usually some sort of change in instruction—even something as simple as "Maybe I could meet with him earlier in the day." Lowering the goal is not considered an appropriate option. Whenever the student achieves four *consecutive* data points above the goal line, the goal is raised (see Fuchs et al., 1989). Using the data in this way allows the teacher to determine if the student is making appropriate progress or if a change in instruction is warranted. If data are not collected frequently, several weeks could go by before these rules could be applied.

The second method, trend line analysis, represents the student's *observed* rate of progress, which can be compared to the *expected* rate of progress as indicated by the goal line. The five steps below describe the Tukey method of trend line analysis.

1. Collect at least seven or eight CBM scores (after establishing the baseline).
2. Divide them as evenly as possible into three groups. For example, if we collected eight data points, we might divide them into the first three, the next two, and the last three.
3. Find the median (middle) score for the first group and the last group and mark them with an X.
4. Draw a line between the two X's.
5. Compare this trend line to the goal line.

Figure 10.6 shows what this process might look like. After 8 weeks of monitoring our student's progress once per week, we have enough data points to draw a trend line. First, we group the first three data points together, the next two, and the last three. Next, we draw an X at the median point of both the first and last three data points. Notice that the X is at the midpoint both vertically (the middle score) and horizontally (the middle time point). The X shouldn't be drawn exactly *on* the middle score unless it occurred at the middle time point for that group. Last, connect the two X's and compare the trend line to the goal line.

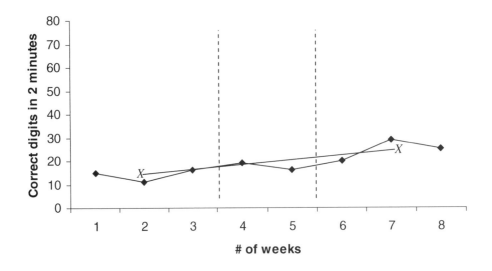

FIGURE 10.6. Example of the Tukey method of drawing a trend line.

If the trend line and goal line are similar, the student is making adequate progress. If the trend line indicates that the student will not be able to reach his goal in the time frame graphed, then instructional changes should be considered. This should be done every seven to eight data points to ensure the student is staying on track. If the trend line is consistently above the goal line, we should consider increasing the goal.

While we provide two ways to review and respond to the data, we would encourage you to use the aim line compared to the goal line as this will provide a more accurate picture of student growth. The best way to determine how a student will perform is to look at past performance. That is why the aim line is the preferred method: it is based on actual student performance projected to the end-of-year performance goal. For a detailed discussion and practical tips on interpreting graphed data, we recommend Riley-Tillman and Burns's (2009) *Evaluating Educational Interventions: Single-Case Design for Measuring Response to Intervention.*

CONSIDERATIONS FOR GRAPHING AND CHARTING THE DATA IN THE CONTENT AREAS

The procedures for graphing are the same no matter in what content area you are monitoring the student's progress. It is possible to use different scales on graphs for different content areas; however, if you are trying to make comparisons across areas, this may make it confusing. For example, the graphs in Figure 10.2 could be for different content areas. Using these two graphs, you could easily draw different conclusions about the student's progress in the different areas, but if you have the student's goal line plotted on each (and you should), you will have a reference point. As such, it may not be a big deal to use different vertical axes for different content areas. We recommend using the same vertical axis for all students in the same content area so that you can make accurate comparisons among students (if you are so inclined) or among grades for the same student. Also keep in mind that if you are graphing errors on the same graph you need to make sure the *Y* axis starts at 0.

THE USE OF CBM IN RTI

You've probably heard of the terms *response to intervention* (RTI) and *multi-tiered system of supports* (MTSS); at the very least, you should have read our brief reference to them in Chapter 1. There are different approaches to RTI/MTSS, but all include the use of data to make decisions about the effectiveness of instruction with students.

RTI/MTSS uses a tiered approach to instruction. Tier 1 is the general instruction provided to all students. Tier 2 adds supplemental instruction for those students who are not making adequate progress with only the Tier 1 instruction. Tier 3 encompasses the most intensive instruction for those students having the greatest difficulties. The same curriculum-based measures are used with all students across the various tiers of instruction; the only thing that really changes is the frequency of assessment. The students who need the most intensive interventions (Tier 3) also need to have their progress monitored most frequently (in addition to universal screening)—one to two times per week. Students receiving supplemental instruction (i.e., Tier 2) would also need to have their progress monitored frequently—once per week. The students making adequate progress with the general instruction (Tier 1) are monitored less frequently—once per month or only using the universal screening assessments three times per year. These data are used to make instructional decisions.

When making decisions, one of the most important parts is to determine an appropriate standard to compare student performance to. Once you have identified the appropriate comparison, you have a basis for making judgments. We have already explained how standards for level of performance and rate of progress can be set for use with CBM. There are benchmarks and if those are not available then norms can be used for performance and progress. These same standards can be used to make two types of decisions within an RTI/MTSS approach.

The first type of decision is about the effectiveness of the instructional program that a student is receiving. If the student's level of performance or rate of progress is below the standard being used, then the instruction is not as effective as we want it to be. The decision we need to make is about how to alter the instruction the student is receiving in order to increase her level of performance or rate of progress. CBM (or any assessment tool) does not give you information specific enough to determine which instructional approach to use or how to alter the current one—this is the time for teachers, as professionals, to use their professional judgment (Hosp et al., 2014). No matter how well developed, an assessment tool does not have the same amount of information about the student as a teacher does. There are some structured approaches to decision making (see the "Resources and/or Further Reading" section of this chapter for some), but they do not tell you what to do—they only provide guidelines for decision making.

The second type of decision made within RTI/MTSS is about eligibility for remedial programs such as special education. Most often, this is mentioned in reference to eligibility for the category of learning disability, but the decision can also be made for a general determination of eligible/not eligible. This is often referred to as a noncategorical approach to special education, since one does not have to determine which disability category a student might belong to before providing services.

The most common method for this approach to eligibility determination is called the *dual discrepancy method*. Because CBM provides you with performance data (the level a student is performing at) and progress data (her rate of growth), you can compare both of these types of data to standards (such as the ones discussed previously in this chapter).

Since this isn't a book on RTI/MTSS, we really can't go into too much detail. Suffice it to say that CBM is a core component of RTI/MTSS. If you are interested in learning more about RTI/MTSS, check out some of the resources listed in the "Resources and/or Further Reading" section of this chapter.

COMPUTERIZED GRAPHING AND DATA MANAGEMENT SYSTEMS

There are many different alternatives for computerized graphing and data management programs. Some are designed to be used specifically with the company's products, and others have the flexibility to incorporate other measures as the user wants. All the programs listed below allow the user to enter and graph data. Some are web-based and some are stand-alone programs (meaning you can install them on a single computer, tablet, or local network). Some programs will also allow for data management and storage over time, which enables cross-year analysis and interpretation. Some will even collect and score the data! Cost for the programs varies. For some it depends on the level of license that is purchased (e.g., individual, schoolwide). For others it depends on which services are purchased. There are three general types of computerized systems: material-specific programs, material-flexible programs, and general spreadsheet and data management programs. It is important to select one that is right for your specific needs. Each program is described in terms of the following criteria:

- *Type*: Is the program web-based (meaning that the data are stored on a remote server and are accessed through the Internet) or stand-alone (meaning that the program is installed on a specific computer and must be accessed through that computer)?
- *Data*: Does the program allow for cross-year data management and analysis, or is it only available for within-year use?
- *Fee*: Is there a fee associated with the program or its use? Is it a one-time fee or an ongoing fee for usage?
- *Auto*: Does the program allow for computerized administration and scoring, or is it solely for data management and interpretation?
- *Skills*: Which skills discussed in this book can be addressed using this program?
- *Note*: This provides additional information about the program (if applicable).

Material-Specific Programs

aimsweb (Pearson: www.aimsweb.com)

- *Type*: web-based
- *Data*: cross-year
- *Fee*: ongoing usage fee
- *Auto*: data management and storage, some browser-based scoring
- *Skills*: Reading, Early Reading, Spelling, Writing, Math, Early Numeracy
- *Note*: Early Reading materials are also available in Spanish.

DIBELS Data System (dibels.uoregon.edu)

- *Type*: web-based
- *Data*: cross-year
- *Fee*: ongoing usage fee
- *Auto*: data management and storage
- *Skills*: Reading, Early Reading, Math, Early Numeracy
- *Note*: Materials are also available in Spanish.

DIBELSnet (dibels.net)

- *Type*: web-based
- *Data*: cross-year
- *Fee*: ongoing usage fee
- *Auto*: data management and storage
- *Skills*: Reading, Early Reading
- *Note*: Materials are also available in Spanish.

EasyCBM (easyCBM.com)

- *Type*: web-based
- *Data*: cross-year
- *Fee*: free (EasyCBM Lite) or with ongoing usage fee
- *Auto*: online administration and scoring (Reading Comprehension, Mathematics), data management and storage
- *Skills*: Reading, Early Reading, Math

Edcheckup (www.edcheckup.com)

- *Type*: web-based
- *Data*: cross-year
- *Fee*: ongoing usage fee
- *Auto*: browser-based scoring, data management and storage
- *Skills*: Reading, Early Reading, Math

FastBridge Learning (fastbridge.org)

- *Type*: web-based
- *Data*: cross-year
- *Fee*: ongoing usage fee
- *Auto*: computerized scoring (OPR only), data management and storage
- *Skills*: Reading, Early Reading, Math, Early Numeracy
- *Note*: Materials are also available in Spanish.

STEEP (isteep.com)

- *Type*: web-based
- *Data*: cross-year
- *Fee*: ongoing usage fee
- *Auto*: online administration (except OPR), scoring, data management, and storage

Yearly Progress Pro (YPP; DRC/CTB: www.ctb.com)

- *Type*: web-based
- *Data*: cross-year
- *Fee*: ongoing usage fee
- *Auto*: computerized administration, scoring, data management, and storage
- *Skills*: Reading (Maze), Math (Computation, Concepts and Applications)

Material-Flexible Program

Intervention Central (Chart Dog: www.interventioncentral.org)

- *Type*: web-based
- *Data*: single year
- *Fee*: none
- *Auto*: data management and storage
- *Skills*: Reading, Early Reading (DIBELS, LSF, WIF), Spelling, Writing, Math (Early Numeracy, Computation, Concepts and Applications)
- *Note*: For progress monitoring only. Can be customized to include any CBM measure.

Spreadsheet and Data Management Programs

DataDirector (Riverside Publishing)

- *Type*: web-based
- *Data*: cross-year
- *Fee*: ongoing usage fee
- *Auto*: data management and storage
- *Note*: Requires more time than using a material-specific system, but has prepopulated reports and formats to meet your needs and save time.

Excel (Microsoft)

- *Type*: stand-alone
- *Data*: cross-year
- *Fee*: one-time fee (comes bundled with Microsoft Office)
- *Auto*: data management and storage
- *Note*: There are some graphs that Excel cannot create; however, data are easily exported into other software that can. Requires more time (due to creating the system from scratch), but is more flexible to meet local needs.

FileMaker Pro (FileMaker)

- *Type*: stand-alone (although there is a web-based version)
- *Data*: cross-year
- *Fee*: one-time fee
- *Auto*: data management and storage
- *Note*: Requires more time (due to creating system from scratch), but is more flexible to meet needs. Not as readily available as Excel (which could create accessibility issues).

Numbers (Apple)

- *Type*: stand-alone
- *Data*: cross-year
- *Fee*: one-time fee
- *Auto*: data management and storage
- *Note*: Requires more time (due to creating system from scratch), but is more flexible to meet needs. Not as readily available as Excel (which could create accessibility issues).

FREQUENTLY ASKED QUESTIONS ABOUT CHARTING AND GRAPHING CBM DATA

1. ***Does the use of CBM lead to changes in students' curriculum?*** CBM doesn't lead to changes in curriculum because that is set by state standards or the student's IEP. It does lead to more frequent changes in instruction, and those changes have been shown to lead to increased student performance. Remember, CBM is not a curriculum or an intervention, but it does provide data on how students are responding to a curriculum or intervention.

2. ***Does the median score reliably predict the student's baseline?*** In general, the median score is considered the baseline. It's not quite the same as in behavior assessment or single-case research, though; it's more like the starting point or a pretreatment score. We can't wait to find a stable baseline over time because we're not measuring skills that should be stable. If a student wasn't improving her performance for 3 or more weeks, we shouldn't be waiting around to try an intervention. We should be panicking.

3. ***If a student reaches his goal early, should I continue to monitor his progress to see if he exceeds the goal?*** Absolutely! You should set a more ambitious goal if the student gets four consecutive scores above his goal line. If the student's goal was to meet a benchmark or catch up to his peers, you could start to monitor his progress less frequently so that you can focus your time on another student having difficulty.

4. ***Why is it important to have intervention lines?*** Intervention lines are put onto the graph in order for you to be able to separate different interventions or phases of the student's instruction more easily. They let you quickly and clearly tell when something different occurred and judge what effect it might have had on the student's rate of progress.

5. *While progress monitoring a student, how many times do you allow her performance to fall below the goal line before reassessing her instructional level?* When a student's performance falls below the goal line for four consecutive data points, you should consider making an instructional change rather than assuming her instructional level is different. Her level of performance is probably fairly stable. It is her rate of progress that is not as good as it should be.

6. *Would it be appropriate to show the student her chart even if her performance is falling below the goal line?* Yes. Students like to see what kind of progress they're making—it can be very motivating when they're doing well and when they're not doing as well as we'd like. Rather than telling the student that she isn't doing well or is failing, the chart can be used to start a discussion about changing instruction (how the discussion goes depends on the student and her grade level). It might start off something like, "You're right. Your progress isn't as good as we want it to be. Maybe we should try something different with how I teach you reading."

7. *When is it appropriate to raise a student's goal?* After collecting a minimum of six to eight data points, a student's goal should be raised when he has four consecutive data points above the goal line.

RESOURCES AND/OR FURTHER READING

Conte, K. L., & Hintze, J. M. (2000). The effects of performance feedback and goal setting on oral reading fluency within curriculum-based measurement. *Diagnostique, 25*(2), 85–98.

Deno, S. L. (1987). Curriculum-based measurement, program development, graphing performance and increasing efficiency. *Teaching Exceptional Children, 20*(1), 41–47.

Graney, S. B. (2008). General education teacher judgments of their low-performing students' short-term reading progress. *Psychology in the Schools, 45*, 537–549.

Jenkins, J., Graff, J., & Miglioretti, D. (2009). Estimating reading growth using intermittent CBM progress monitoring. *Exceptional Children, 75*, 151–163.

Jenkins, J., & Terjeson, K. (2011). Monitoring reading growth: Goal setting, measurement frequency, and methods of evaluation. *Learning Disabilities: Research and Practice, 26*, 28–35.

Jimerson, S., Burns, M., & VanDerHeyden, A. (Eds.). (2016). *Handbook of response to intervention: The science and practice of assessment and intervention* (2nd ed.). New York: Springer.

National Association of School Psychologists. (2006). *Assessment alternatives under IDEA 2004* (CD-ROM Toolkit). Bethesda, MD: Author.

Riley-Tillman, T., & Burns, M. (2009). *Evaluating educational interventions: Single-case designs for measuring response to intervention*. New York: Guilford Press.

Shinn, M. R. (1989). Identifying and defining academic problems: CBM screening and eligibility procedures. In M. R. Shinn (Ed.), *Curriculum-based measurement: Assessing special children* (pp. 94–99). New York: Guilford Press.

CHAPTER 11

Planning to Use CBM— and Keeping It Going

Our best intentions will not go far without a solid plan for carrying them out. It is worth putting in the time and effort up front to ensure successful implementation of CBM. Getting it going is only half of it, though; planning how to keep it going is the other half and just as important. We would also stress that collecting data for the sake of collecting data should be avoided at all costs. What is done with the data is what will ultimately make the difference for a student. Therefore, we encourage people to use a process like CBE to help determine next steps and helpful ways to review and use the data to make better instructional decisions. Please see Chapter 2 for further information related to how CBE and CBM fit together. In this chapter, we outline ways to help plan for using CBM before, during, and after initial implementation. We also offer helpful hints on how to get and keep CBM going. We would encourage people to also use the CBE process to help guide use of the data once they are collected.

DEVELOPING A PLAN FOR USING CBM

So you have decided to implement CBM. Congratulations! With a well-developed plan you will soon see how CBM will allow you to help all students achieve greater success in school. This is possible because CBM provides a database for each student that allows you to evaluate the effectiveness of the instruction he or she is receiving. Whether you are looking at implementing CBM at the classroom, grade, schoolwide, or district level, the factors that need to be considered will be similar.

We have broken the task of planning to use CBM into 10 steps. In Appendix B we provide a checklist to get you started. Below are points to consider to ensure you are making informed decisions as you complete the checklist.

Ten Steps to Using CBM before, during, and after Initial Implementation

Before

STEP 1: WHO WILL BE USING CBM?

This depends on what it will be used for. The following are some points to consider for each level of use:

- *Classroom(s)*: Is this something only one teacher is interested in? If yes, then this teacher will be able to screen and track the progress of her class, but she will not be able to have a conversation with her same-grade colleagues about how they are doing as a whole grade to meet the needs of all of their students.

- *Grade(s)*: Is this something only one grade is interested in? If yes, the teachers in that grade will be able to screen and track progress for all of their students, but they will not be able to learn how the students in their grade compare to other grades in that school or other schools in that district.

- *School(s)*: Is this something only one school is interested in? If yes, teachers in that school will be able to screen and track progress for all of their students. They will be able to look across grades and see how many students are proficient and making progress in a given year and across years. This provides a good overall indication of how the students are achieving in the school, but if only one or two schools use CBM, then they will not be able to compare how their students are doing with others in the district.

- *District*: Is the district deciding to adopt CBM for every school? If yes, teachers in that district will be able to screen and track the progress of every student enrolled. They will be able to look at the entire system to determine if all grades are meeting the needs of the students based on how many students are at benchmark on universal screening. This provides a districtwide view but can also be broken down by building, grade, classroom, and subgroups. When CBM data are available for every student, there are many more questions that can be asked and answered. One word of caution is that every school in the district needs to be using similar materials and assessing students during the same time period in order to be able to make comparisons.

STEP 2: WHICH CBM SKILLS WILL BE IMPLEMENTED?

This may be a hard question to answer if you are interested in all the areas of CBM. Since the majority of student problems in school are in the area of reading, this might be a good place to start. The following are some points to consider for each area:

- *Early reading* (onset sounds, phoneme segmenting, letter naming, letter sounds, nonsense words, word identification): Skill level of students is important to consider—some early reading skills are not needed for students who have already mastered them. However, never assume they have mastered them without first having data to support that assumption.

- *Reading* (OPR, maze passage reading): Only Maze CBM can be administered to a group, but reading is a critical area, and these measures are great for universal screening and progress monitoring.

- *Spelling*: Can be administered to a group, which saves time.

- *Writing*: Is the longest CBM measure to implement, but can be administered to a group, which saves time. It would be a great add-on once one of the other areas is going strong.

- *Early Numeracy* (oral counting, touch counting, number identification, missing number, quantity discrimination): These are all designed to be given individually.

- *Math* (computation [mixed operation and single operation], concepts and applications): Can be administered to a group, which saves time.

- *Vocabulary:* Can be administered to a group, which saves time.

STEP 3: WHAT MATERIALS WILL WE USE?

This is a very important decision that will make the process either easy or hard. The following are some points to consider for each area:

- *Use a commercial product with scoring and graphing capabilities*: These can be a real time saver as well as offering some of the better products out there. These programs are usually web-based, meaning that the assessments can be given anywhere and the data can be viewed from anywhere. The data can be looked at by the individual student, teachers, principals, and other administrators. In some cases, parents can get online access to their child's data.

- *Purchase premade material and make your own graphing program*: This option is probably best if just one or two teachers are going to be using CBM. The downside is that you have to photocopy and organize the material as well as build and run your own graphing program. Sources for obtaining premade material are provided in text boxes in Chapters 3–9.

- *Purchase premade material and graph on paper*: This option is probably only reasonable for the single teacher who will be using CBM only for his class or for a few students.

STEP 4: WHEN WILL IMPLEMENTATION START?

Timing is everything, so it is important to plan as far ahead as possible. One thing to remember is that you will need a few weeks to prepare for training, ordering and getting the materials together, and practicing. The following are some points to consider for each time of year:

- *Fall*: This is the best time to start with universal screening and progress monitoring. This will mean planning at the end of the previous year or over the summer before students arrive. It is important to wait a couple of weeks before testing to allow the students to regain some skills they may have not been using or practicing over the long summer break.

- *Winter*: If training, materials, and organization don't come together in the fall, then waiting until winter may be a better plan than rushing, only to have things done incorrectly. You can still screen all students and start progress monitoring in the winter; you will just not have the benefit of the fall data for this first year. The testing window should not follow directly after a long break, but should be planned so students have time to get back into their learning routines.

- *Spring*: This is the last choice for when to start; however, the spring could be used to introduce staff to CBM, conduct some training, and practice giving the measures. If you use this model, you will want to make sure that a review training is also included in the fall, since there will be a period of time during which staff will not have used the measures.

STEP 5: WHO WILL TRAIN THE STAFF?

The message sometimes is only as good as the messenger. We have seen the best of practices implemented poorly due to poor training. It is usually worth the money to make sure the training is done well and at the level of sophistication the staff needs to support their learning. The following are some points to consider for each option:

- *Hire a professional trainer to train the staff*: Not all professional training is equal, so ask around and try to use people who have expertise and can provide excellent training. If resources are an issue, then try to coordinate these efforts with other schools and possibly other districts nearby. Good training can make all the difference. Along these lines, follow-up training should also be built into the plan. Having someone come back and help troubleshoot as well as assist with interpreting the data is well worth it.

- *Have a couple of staff members receive professional training and then train the rest of the staff*: This can save time and expense and work well if the staff members being trained already have a strong knowledge base in CBM. If not, the information shared may not be a true representation of how to conduct CBM.

- *Train yourselves by using published materials and practicing together as a group*: If professional training is not an option, then getting a group together to learn and practice the materials may be the way to go. One caution is that the group should already have some knowledge of assessment and understand the importance of standardized directions. More time to learn and practice will need to be built into this model so that when CBM is conducted it is done correctly.

During

STEP 6: WHO WILL MANAGE THE MATERIALS?

This is an organization and time-management issue. Managing the materials can include purchasing, printing and collating, distributing, storing, putting student names on materials, or adding students into an online data system. The person responsible for managing the material needs to have time allocated for this task. It takes time to purchase or print material and organize it for every teacher and student. It is best to organize the material well in advance so that things can be double-checked. This also allows for time to practice administering and scoring the measures prior to collecting data. The following are some points to consider for each option:

- *Teacher* (general education, Title I, ESL, special education): Having an individual teacher manage the materials can be a smart way to go, since teachers are already familiar with the details that go into testing students. They are often better at thinking up strategies to improve the efficiency of making, collecting, and storing materials. If only one person is responsible for managing the online database, this can also limit the number of errors that can occur from having too many people with editing rights.

- *Administrator* (principal, vice principal): Having an administrator manage the materials is a nice way to involve him or her in the process, but most administrators have schedules that prohibit them from managing the materials on a day-to-day basis. It might be better to include administrators in the training and possibly in the collection of data.

- *Support staff* (speech therapist, reading specialist, school psychologist): Having support staff manage the materials can be a good way to get them involved and working directly with the other educators in the school. One problem is that support staff may not always be in your building, making it hard to reach them at times.

- *Assistant* (administrative assistants, parent volunteers): Having an administrative assistant or parent volunteer may be a good choice if they have the time and organizational skills. With any volunteer, you want to be careful about confidentiality issues related to students' work.

STEP 7: WHO WILL COLLECT THE DATA?

This is critical to the time it will take to collect the data as well as who has ownership of it. Time spent and ownership of the data are the two main issues that should guide you when making a plan. In addition, making sure the data are collected with fidelity is critical. See the General Fidelity Checklist for Conducting CBM in Appendix B to assist with this. The following are some points to consider for each option:

- *Individual teachers*: Having teachers help with data collection allows them to learn CBM and have an understanding of the tasks the student is asked to perform and what the results mean. Our experience has been that if teachers do not collect the data for their own students, they may view them as "your data" and not "their data." When it comes to progress monitoring, teachers should collect the data for their own students. When conducting universal screening, it may be more efficient to use a team approach where the teacher helps collect some of the data in her class but is not responsible for the collection of all the data. However, if teachers can collect the data on all of their students, this is preferred, as it can provide them with information they would not otherwise have.

- *Teams* (general and special education teachers, educational assistants, principals, school psychologists, reading specialists, speech therapists): This is a great approach to use when collecting data for universal screening. The more people at the school or district who are trained, the faster the data collection will go. It also shows that people value what is happening enough to get involved and help out. This is especially true if the principal joins in. A word of caution about using parent volunteers and older students to help collect the data. We have found that confidentiality can be jeopardized by including people who are not directly employed by the school. Also, parents and older students often do not have the expertise in assessment to ensure the data are collected correctly.

STEP 8: WHERE WILL THE DATA BE COLLECTED?

This is also a time-management issue. Data collection should be done in the most efficient way that will provide the least amount of disruption to teaching while allowing the data to be collected quickly. The following are some points to consider for each location:

- *In the classroom*: This can be done by having the individual teacher assess all of her own students. This takes time away from teaching, however, and may not be the fastest way to collect the data. A team could go into the classroom and help assess all of the students. While this may not take as much time away from teaching, it may not be the fastest way to collect the data because the team would have to organize each classroom separately as well as bring all of the materials with them.

- *Central location* (library, cafeteria, multipurpose room): This takes little time away from teaching and is the best way to collect all the data quickly. A team would only have to organize one room, as they would have all of their material in one place and could move through classrooms of students rather quickly. One way to speed this process up is to have classrooms come to the central location as a group. While some students are being assessed, others can be kept busy reading a book silently while being supervised. This is where parent volunteers and other staff can help out by supervising those students waiting and bringing in the next class when the team is ready.

After

STEP 9: WHO WILL MANAGE THE DATA ONCE THEY ARE COLLECTED?

There are simple ways to manage the data that will make using CBM time and energy efficient. This step, like all of the others, is critical to the success of using any type of assessment. With the development of more online CBM databases and materials, the task of managing the data has been streamlined and is becoming much more efficient. Online data systems allow the teacher to enter the responses in real time and then automatically score, graph, and store the data as soon as the assessment is completed. This time savings adds to the efficiency of data collection and allows more time for teachers to review and discuss the data. The following are some points to consider for each option:

- *Each teacher is responsible for entering and graphing her students' data*: This is not a bad idea if this time can be planned for and built into teachers' schedules. It would allow for a quick turnaround time from when students are assessed to when graphs are printed. It is not necessarily the task of entering and graphing that makes the difference, however, but rather the act of looking at the data and planning instruction. Therefore, it is not always necessary for teachers to do this. Online CBM programs would allow for every teacher to do this efficiently.

• *One person for each grade or school is responsible for entering and graphing the data*: This may be more time efficient if there are people at each school who could have this task built into their duties. This means they would have to have times where they would be available to enter the data and print graphs. Having one or more people to do this assigned at each school may decrease the turnaround time from when the students are assessed to when the data are entered and graphs printed.

• *A team of people at the district is responsible for entering and graphing the data*: Having someone at the district level perform this task would be the last resort. If the data need to be moved to another location to be entered and then the graphs have to be brought back to each school, this could increase the time lag between assessing the students and getting the information back. It is not a bad idea, however, to have someone at the district level who understands the assessment and can assist in reading and interpreting the data.

STEP 10: HOW WILL THE DATA BE SHARED?

If the data are collected, entered, graphed, and printed but then put into a drawer, they may as well not have been collected at all. This holds true whether you use an online program or enter the data by hand into a graphing program. A wise principal once told us "Out of sight is out of mind. I want my teachers looking at their data every day." This last step closes the circle and makes the process whole. Having an administrator participate in the data discussions is also helpful when making decisions about instruction at a grade or district level. The following are some points to consider for data sharing:

• *Each teacher is responsible for looking at her data by herself*: If only one teacher in the school is using CBM, then this is OK, but otherwise it is more efficient and effective to have teachers working together to determine what the data mean as well as identifying interventions to use.

• *At the grade level, all of the teachers look at all of the students together*: This is a great way for the teachers in each grade to look at an entire grade, as well as groups of students and individual students who may need additional help. A team approach is always preferred over a single person when looking at the data.

• *At the school level, a team is responsible for looking at all of the students*: This may be time efficient, but if the team members are not familiar with the students, they may have a harder time understanding what to do about individual students. Looking at the grade levels to identify trends and possible areas of weakness in the curriculum would be appropriate at this level.

HINTS ON HOW TO GET CBM GOING

There are many ways to approach getting CBM going in a classroom, grade, school, or district. The most effective way is to have a team of people, including someone from the administration, such as a principal, a district coordinator for assessment or special services, or even a superintendent. Other members could be general education or special education teachers and specialists like reading coaches, speech therapists, school psychologists, or counselors. We have found implementation and sustainability to be greater with a group of people working together for a common goal.

This team can educate others on some of the reasons to use CBM. The following list provides some ideas and pointers to use.

- It is fast and efficient to administer and score.
- It provides excellent information on students' overall skills in reading, spelling, writing, and math.
- It is fluency based.
- It allows for more time teaching and less time assessing.
- It can be used to group students and help plan instruction.
- It can be used to look at general trends across grades.
- It can be used to screen all students at least three times per year.
- It allows for progress monitoring throughout the year in a quick and easy manner.
- It is a reliable and valid measure of students' skills that has more than 30 years of research behind it.
- It could replace other more costly and lengthy tests.
- It can be graphed so the data are easy to share with students and parents.

HINTS ON HOW TO KEEP CBM GOING

Planning ahead and being prepared for questions is one way to ensure that CBM will become a standard in a school or district. It will take work to keep it going. Below we provide a list of activities and ideas that can help.

- *Prepare the materials ahead of time for the entire year*: This would include materials needed to screen and progress monitor. Here are some tips: Color-code student books by grades so they are easy to identify when testing multiple grades. Having the students' names printed on labels and placed on the materials can also save a lot of time. Make extra copies of student materials for retesting or in case additional students move into the district. Another tip is to have the teacher/examiner materials laminated or put in pocket protectors and into a binder so that they are easy to locate and will have sustainability over the years. If you are using an online system, allow time to upload student information and make sure the system is working as intended before starting testing.

• *Have a schedule planned before the year starts*: Putting dates down on a calendar for the entire year will help everyone plan when universal screening will occur, when progress monitoring will happen, and when data will be shared and discussed. You can easily remind everyone about what is happening by distributing a monthly calendar (or adding these things to the school monthly calendar that is already developed) with the CBM information specific to that month. Here are two tips to consider. One is to incorporate the collection of progress monitoring data throughout the week rather than stopping instruction for an entire day to collect progress monitoring data. We have actually seen this in many schools where one person is responsible for the progress monitoring data and spends one day a week just testing students. Instead, each student's teacher should be collecting the data so he or she can see the progress of his or her student and better understand how best to help that student. Another tip is to wait at least 2 instructional weeks after any long break before conducting assessments (especially universal screening). Some students need time after a break to get back in the swing of things, and if we assess them too early, they will not have the opportunity to show us their best skills.

• *Incorporate the data into everyday use*: The data could be brought to weekly grade-level meetings, and any students who are struggling could be discussed. Another way to incorporate the data is to send home weekly progress monitoring sheets to parents so they can see how their children are doing. This information could also be shared at parent–teacher conferences. The scores could be incorporated on the students' report cards.

• *Regularly share successes with colleagues*: This could take place at weekly or monthly staff or grade-level meetings. A more formal way to do this would be to put out a newsletter that highlights the successes of CBM throughout the district or school.

• *Conduct follow-up or review sessions when needed*: Especially during the first year, it will be helpful to have review sessions that allow staff to ask questions as they become more familiar with the assessment procedures. It might be helpful to hire a consultant to assist with this if there is currently no one on staff who is qualified or experienced enough to answer these questions.

• *Rotate the management of data collection so the person in charge does not get burned out*: This will also give others an opportunity to learn additional skills when collecting and using CBM data. One suggestion would be to rotate from grade to grade each quarter, half year, or year. Using an online system will help prevent burnout as these systems are more efficient for everyone to use.

FREQUENTLY ASKED QUESTIONS ABOUT PLANNING AND USING CBM

1. *As a special educator, will I be allowed to use CBM if the school doesn't use it?* Yes. If you write your IEP goals and objectives using CBM data, you will not only be allowed to use CBM but required to. Special educators need to monitor all of their students closely.

CBM allows you to do this in a timely and efficient manner so that you can determine which students are responding to your instruction and which are not.

2. *How can I persuade my school to adopt CBM or at least allow me to use it?* None of us has met an administrator who has said "no" when asked, "If I can track students' progress every week using an assessment that is reliable and valid and will only take me 1–5 minutes per student, would you say 'yes'?" Another way to sell it is to show the administrator the graphs and how you will track progress toward goals that will inform you, the student, the administrator, and the parents.

3. *Can anyone administer CBM assessments? Can a paraprofessional give them?* There are people we would recommend and not recommend for administering CBM assessments; however, it should be possible to train and supervise anyone who works at a school so that they can help collect CBM data. People we do not recommend using are parent volunteers and students due to confidentiality issues and reliability in administering and scoring the assessments.

4. *Would it be a good idea to involve the parents of a struggling student by having them also conduct CBM at home, or should it only be done in the classroom?* The data collection should only be conducted by one person to ensure the reliability and accuracy of the data collected. Therefore, we would recommend having only the teacher administer CBM. It is a great idea to involve parents by sending home the student graphs on a weekly basis and encouraging parents to have their children read aloud to them. If you also want parents to collect CBM data, you should provide them with their own CBM graph to use, while you keep yours at school.

5. *Which CBM task should I use if this is my first time using CBM?* We would recommend reading as probably the best task to start with. It could be Early Reading CBM, OPR CBM, or Maze CBM. The reason is that reading is the most critical skill students need to be proficient in to be successful in school and life. Curriculum-based measures for reading also have the most research behind their use and are widely available from multiple sources.

RESOURCES AND/OR FURTHER READING

Allinder, R. M. (1996). When some is not better than none: Effects of differential implementation of curriculum-based measurement. *Exceptional Children, 62,* 525–535.

Allinder, R. M., & BeckBest, M. A. (1995). Differential effects of two approaches to supporting teachers' use of curriculum-based measurement. *School Psychology Review, 24,* 287–298.

Burns, M. K. (2002). Comprehensive system of assessment to intervention using curriculum-based assessments. *Intervention in School and Clinic, 38*(1), 8–13.

Fuchs, L. S., & Fuchs, D. (1993). Effects of systematic observation and feedback on teachers' implementation of curriculum-based measurement. *Teacher Education and Special Education, 16,* 178–187.

Hasbrouck, J. E., Woldbeck, T., Ihnot, C., & Parker, R. I. (1999). One teacher's use of curriculum-based measurement: A changed opinion. *Learning Disabilities Research and Practice, 14,* 118–126.

Howe, K. B., Scierka, B. J., Gibbons, K. A., & Silberglitt, B. (2003). A schoolwide organization system for raising reading achievement using general outcome measures and evidence-based instruction: One education district's experience. *Assessment for Effective Intervention, 28*(3/4), 59–71.

Marston, D. B., & Magnusson, D. (1985). Implementing curriculum-based measurement in special and regular education settings. *Exceptional Children, 52,* 266–276.

Rowe, S. S., Witner, S., Cook, E., & DaCruz, K. (2014). Teachers' attitudes about using curriculum-based measurement in reading (CBM-R) for universal screening and progress monitoring. *Journal of Applied School Psychology, 30,* 305–337.

Whinnery, K. W., & Fuchs, L. S. (1992). Implementing effective teaching strategies with learning disabled students through curriculum-based measurement. *Learning Disabilities Research and Practice, 7*(1), 25–30.

Yell, M. L., Deno, S. L., & Marston, D. B. (1992). Barriers to implementing curriculum-based measurement. *Diagnostique, 18*(1), 99–112.

Norms for Early Reading CBM, OPR CBM, and Maze CBM

We provide norm tables here for some of the reading curriculum-based measures and have included benchmarks within Chapters 3 and 4 (for Early Reading CBM and Reading CBM, respectively). All other norm tables—for Spelling CBM, Writing CBM, Early Numeracy CBM, and Math CBM—are provided within Chapters 5, 6, 7, and 8, respectively, since there are no benchmarks available.

TABLE A1. Norms for Early Reading CBM

Percentile	Kindergarten			Grade 1		
	Fall	Winter	Spring	Fall	Winter	Spring
Onset Sounds						
90%	16	16	16	—	—	—
75%	15	16	16	—	—	—
50%	**13**	**16**	**16**	—	—	—
25%	9	14	16	—	—	—
10%	6	12	15	—	—	—
Phoneme Segmenting/ Word Segmenting						
90%	19	32	34	33	34	34
75%	10	30	32	31	33	34
50%	**5**	**26**	**30**	**28**	**30**	**32**
25%	0	19	27	24	27	30
10%	0	10	22	19	24	27
Letter Names						
90%	45	64	70	62	75	—
75%	38	55	60	52	69	—
50%	**25**	**45**	**52**	**44**	**59**	—
25%	14	36	43	36	48	—
10%	5	26	35	28	39	—
Letter Sounds						
90%	31	49	61	49	65	—
75%	23	42	53	43	56	—
50%	**13**	**33**	**44**	**33**	**47**	—
25%	5	23	36	25	36	—
10%	1	15	27	19	23	—
Nonsense Words						
90%	—	14	21	22	33	42
75%	—	11	17	16	24	32
50%	—	**7**	**13**	**11**	**17**	**23**
25%	—	4	9	7	12	16
10%	—	1	5	4	9	12
Word Identification/ Sight Words						
90%	—	40	58	62	80	93
75%	—	20	44	49	67	82
50%	—	**8**	**25**	**27**	**52**	**69**
25%	—	4	11	11	35	56
10%	—	1	5	5	21	44

Note. Reprinted with permission from FastBridge Learning.

TABLE A2. Norms for OPR CBM: Words Read Correctly (WRC)

Grade	Percentile	Fall (WRC)	Winter (WRC)	Spring (WRC)
1	90%	67	100	128
	75%	31	68	97
	50%	**13**	**36**	**67**
	25%	6	19	40
	10%	2	11	22
2	90%	115	140	156
	75%	88	115	131
	50%	**62**	**88**	**106**
	25%	35	64	82
	10%	17	39	59
3	90%	143	162	179
	75%	116	139	152
	50%	**87**	**111**	**127**
	25%	59	84	98
	10%	38	56	73
4	90%	160	178	196
	75%	134	152	168
	50%	**107**	**125**	**139**
	25%	84	101	112
	10%	61	78	90
5	90%	176	192	205
	75%	150	168	181
	50%	**121**	**139**	**153**
	25%	94	111	123
	10%	74	87	98
6	90%	189	204	219
	75%	165	179	195
	50%	**141**	**155**	**166**
	25%	116	131	141
	10%	91	106	115
7	90%	188	199	213
	75%	167	180	190
	50%	**144**	**155**	**167**
	25%	119	130	141
	10%	97	107	118
8	90%	184	194	203
	75%	165	175	185
	50%	**146**	**155**	**163**
	25%	123	132	142
	10%	99	109	119

Note. From aimsweb (2015).

TABLE A3. Norms for Maze CBM: Words Correctly Restored (WCR)

Grade	Percentile	Fall (WCR)	Winter (WCR)	Spring (WCR)
1	90%	6	14	17
	75%	3	9	13
	50%	**1**	**4**	**8**
	25%	1	2	5
	10%	0	1	2
2	90%	12	21	24
	75%	8	16	20
	50%	**4**	**11**	**15**
	25%	2	6	10
	10%	1	4	7
3	90%	22	25	28
	75%	17	20	22
	50%	**13**	**15**	**16**
	25%	8	11	11
	10%	5	7	8
4	90%	22	32	34
	75%	18	27	28
	50%	**14**	**20**	**20**
	25%	10	15	15
	10%	6	11	11
5	90%	29	35	39
	75%	23	29	33
	50%	**17**	**22**	**27**
	25%	12	17	20
	10%	8	12	15
6	90%	36	43	44
	75%	28	35	35
	50%	**22**	**29**	**28**
	25%	16	22	22
	10%	11	17	16
7	90%	37	40	45
	75%	31	33	39
	50%	**24**	**27**	**31**
	25%	18	20	24
	10%	14	15	18
8	90%	38	37	44
	75%	31	29	36
	50%	**25**	**23**	**28**
	25%	18	17	22
	10%	13	13	17

Note. From aimsweb (2015).

Reproducible Quick Guides and Forms for Conducting CBM

Chapter 6

Chapter 7

Chapter 8

Chapter 9

Chapter 10

Chapter 11

QUICK ADMINISTRATION GUIDE FOR ONSET SOUNDS CBM

1. Place the Onset Sounds CBM practice copy with the four pictures in front of the student. There are five pages total (one practice, four test pages). Place the remaining test pages face down beside the teacher/examiner.

2. Place the teacher/examiner copy on the clipboard or pull up the scoring sheet on the computer screen so the student cannot see it.

3. Say: *"We will do an activity with word sounds. Look at these pictures. This is a key, bat, dolphin, and water* (point to each picture as you say the word). *Which one of these words begins with the /k/ sound—'key,' 'bat,' 'dolphin,' or 'water'?"*
   a. If correct, say: *"Good. 'Key' begins with /k/"* and move to practice item 2.
   b. If incorrect, say: *"Let's try again. 'Key'* (point to the key) *begins with /k/. /k/—'key.'* (Remove your finger from the picture.) *Which one of these words begins with /k/?"*
   c. If correct, say: *"Good, 'key' begins with /k/"* (point to the key).
   d. If incorrect, say: *"'Key' begins with /k/"* (point to the key) and move to extra practice 1.

(continued on other side)

---

4. For practice item 2, say: *"Let's try something different. This time, I'll say the word and then you give the first sound.* (Point to the bat.) *'Bat.' The first sound in the word 'bat' is /b/. Now you try. What is the first sound in the word 'water'?"* (Point to the picture of water.)
   a. If correct, say: *"Good. 'Water' begins with /w/"* and move to begin test.
   b. If incorrect, say: *"Let's try again. 'Water'* (point to the water) *begins with /w/. /w/—'water.' What is the first sound in the word 'water'?* (point to the water). *Remember, just tell the sound."*
   c. If correct, say: *"Good, 'water' begins with /w/."*
   d. If incorrect, say: *"Listen, 'water' begins with /w/. The first sound is /w/"* and begin test.

5. To begin test, say: *"I will show you more pictures. Remember to listen to the names of the pictures and answer each question. Let's begin."* (Start timer.)

6. Place the first Onset Sounds test sheet with the four pictures in front of the student. Ask each question clearly and point to each picture as you say the word. Once a student responds, ask the next question immediately. Do not give any more feedback about the student's response. If the student pauses for 5 seconds without responding to an item, count the item incorrect and continue with the next item. Continue through item 16 using prompts provided on the FastBridge Learning assessment page.

7. Stop timer after item 16 is completed or if test is discontinued.

Adapted with permission from FastBridge Learning.

QUICK SCORING GUIDE FOR ONSET SOUNDS CBM

Scored as Correct

Onset Sounds CBM is scored based on the correct production or identification of the initial sound(s). Each correct initial sound is marked as correct (1) on the score sheet.

Pronounced correctly: The first sound or sounds are pronounced correctly.

Answered correctly: The correct picture is pointed to that corresponds to the sound given.

Self-corrections within 5 seconds: Words mispronounced initially but corrected within 5 seconds and pictures pointed to incorrectly but corrected within 5 seconds.

Dialect/articulation: Variations in pronunciation explainable by local language norms or speech sound production.

Repetitions: Repeating the sound or pointing to the stimuli more than once.

Insertions: Adding the schwa sound.

Scored as Errors

All errors are marked by checking incorrect (0) on the score sheet.

Mispronunciations/substitutions: When a sound is said incorrectly or is substituted with another sound or when the incorrect stimulus is pointed to.

Hesitations without response: Not responding for 5 seconds and being prompted by having the next question read.

Hesitations with response: Starting to respond but not finishing by 5 seconds and being prompted by having the next question read.

QUICK ADMINISTRATION GUIDE FOR PHONEME SEGMENTING CBM

1. Place the teacher/examiner copy on the clipboard so the student cannot see it.
2. Say: *"We are going to say the sounds in words. Listen to me say all the sounds in the word 'fan': /f/ /a/ /n/. Listen to another word* (pause)*: 'jump': /j/ /u/ /m/ /p/. Your turn. Say all the sounds in 'soap.'"*
   a. If correct, say: *"Very good saying all the sounds in 'soap.'"* Begin testing.
   b. If incorrect, say: *"I said 'soap,' so you say /s/ /oa/ /p/. Your turn. Say all the sounds in 'soap.'"*
   c. If correct, say: *"Good."* Begin testing.
   d. If incorrect, say: *"OK."* Begin testing.
3. To begin testing, say: *"I am going to say more words. I will say the word and you say all the sounds in the word."*
4. Say the first word on the list and then start the timer.
5. Stop the timer after 1 minute and put a bracket after the last sound the student says.

———
Adapted with permission from DIBELS.

QUICK SCORING GUIDE FOR PHONEME SEGMENTING CBM

Scored as Correct

Phoneme Segmenting CBM is scored based on each different correct part of the word that is said. Each correct part is underlined and counted as a correct sound segment.

Pronounced correctly: Each sound segment is pronounced correctly.

Self-corrections within 3 seconds: Segments mispronounced initially but corrected within 3 seconds.

Dialect/articulation: Variations in pronunciation explainable by local language norms or speech sound production.

Repetitions: Repeating the same sound more than once.

Insertions: Adding sounds to the beginning, middle, or end of the word or the schwa sound.

Scored as Errors

All errors are marked by drawing a line through the mispronounced sound(s). Sounds that are not produced are left blank. If the student does not segment the word, the word is circled.

Mispronunciations/substitutions: When a sound is said incorrectly or substituted with another sound.

Omissions: Sounds that are not produced.

Hesitations without response: Not responding for 3 seconds and being prompted by having the next word read.

Hesitations with response: Starting to respond but not finishing by 3 seconds and being prompted by having the next word read.

Reversals: Transposing two or more sounds.

Read as whole word: Not segmenting the word into different parts.

QUICK ADMINISTRATION GUIDE FOR LETTER NAMING CBM

1. Place the copy of the student sheet in front of the student.
2. Place the teacher/examiner copy on the clipboard so the student cannot see it.
3. Say: *"I am going to show you some letters. I want you to point to each letter and say its name."* (*Put the page of letters in front of the student.*)
4. To begin testing say: *"Start here* (*point to the first letter at the top of the page*). *Go this way* (*sweep your finger across the first two rows of letters*) *and say each letter name. Put your finger under the first letter* (*point*). *Ready, begin."*
5. Start the timer after you say: *"Begin."*
6. Stop the timer after 1 minute and bracket the last letter named.

———

Adapted with permission from DIBELS.

QUICK SCORING GUIDE FOR LETTER NAMING CBM

Scored as Correct

Letter Naming CBM is scored based on each correct pronunciation of the individual names of the letters. Each correct letter is counted toward total correct letter names; only errors and self-corrections are marked on the sheet.

Pronounced correctly: Each letter must be named correctly.

Self-corrections within 3 seconds: Letter names mispronounced initially but corrected within 3 seconds.

Dialect/articulation: Variations in pronunciation explainable by local language norms or speech sound production.

Repetitions: Repeating the letter name more than once.

Scored as Errors

All errors are marked by drawing a line through the mispronounced or skipped letter.

Mispronunciations/Substitution: When a letter is named incorrectly.

Omissions: Letters that are not produced.

Hesitations without response: Not responding for 3 seconds and being prompted by providing the name of that letter.

Hesitations with response: Starting to respond but not finishing by 3 seconds and being prompted by providing the name of that letter.

Reversals: Transposing two or more letters.

┌───┐

QUICK SCORING GUIDE FOR LETTER SOUNDS CBM

Scored as Correct

Letter Sounds CBM is scored based on pronouncing the most common sound of the letter correctly. Each correct sound is counted toward total correct letter sounds; only errors are marked on the sheet. A pronunciation key for the most common sounds is provided in Table 3.2.

Pronounced correctly: The sound must be pronounced correctly. Short vowel (not long vowel) sounds are considered correct.

Self-corrections within 3 seconds: Sounds mispronounced initially but corrected within 3 seconds are scored as correct and *sc* is written above the letter.

Dialect/articulation: Variations in pronunciation explainable by local language norms or speech sound production.

Repetitions: Repeating the sound more than once.

Insertions: Adding the schwa sound.

Scored as Errors

All errors are marked by drawing a line through the misprounced or skipped letter.

Mispronunciations/substitutions: When a letter sound is either mispronounced or substituted with other letter sounds.

Omissions: Letter sounds that are not produced.

Hesitations without response: Not responding for 3 seconds and being prompted by providing the sound of that letter.

Reversals: Transposing two or more sounds.

└───┘

QUICK ADMINISTRATION GUIDE FOR NONSENSE WORDS CBM

1. Place the copy of the practice page in front of the student.

2. Place the teacher/examiner copy on the clipboard or pull up the scoring sheet on the computer screen so the student cannot see it.

3. Say: *"I am going to have you read some pretend words. An example of a pretend word is 'tup'* (point to the word "tup"). *If you cannot say the word, you can say the sounds in the word: /t/ /u/ /p/* (point to each letter in the word). *When you read these words, try to say the whole word. If you don't know how to say it, then you can say the sounds of each letter instead."*

4. Say: *"Now you try. Read this pretend word"* (point to "pof").
   a. If the student reads as whole word, say: *"Good! The letters 'P', 'O', and 'F' make the pretend word 'POF.'"* Begin directions for test.
   b. If the student reads the sounds, say: *"Good! The letter sounds in 'POF' are /p/ /o/ /f/."* Begin directions for test.
   c. If incorrect, say: *"The pretend word is 'POF': /p/ /o/ /f/—'POF.' When you say the sounds together the pretend word is 'POF.' The sounds in 'POF' are /p/ /o/ /f/. Remember you can say the individual letter sounds OR the whole word."* Begin directions for test.

(continued on other side)

---

5. To begin the test say: *"Now here is a list of more pretend words for you to read. When I say 'Begin' start reading the pretend words out loud here* (point to the first word). *Read across the page, then go to the next line* (point to demonstrate). *Try to say each one as a whole word. If you can't say it as a whole word, then try to sound out the letters."*

6. Say: *"OK? So what are you going to do?"* (Have the student tell you how she can say the whole nonsense word OR the sounds in the words—not both. Clarify if needed). *"Good."*

7. Say: *"Ready? Begin."* (Start timer when student says the first nonsense word.)

8. Follow along on the teacher/examiner copy and click on words that are said incorrectly if using the computer version, or for the paper/pencil version put a slash (/) through any incorrect nonsense words. (The test is not scored at the sound level, so if the student is reading it sound for sound the entire word is still the unit for scoring purposes.)

9. At the end of 1 minute say *"Stop"* and put a bracket (]) after the last word read.

Adapted with permission from FastBridge Learning.

QUICK SCORING GUIDE FOR NONSENSE WORDS CBM

Scored as Correct

Nonsense Words CBM is scored based on pronouncing the most common sound of the letter correctly either letter-by-letter or blended together and read as an entire word. Vowel sounds: Short vowel (not long vowel) sounds are considered correct along with the most common sound for the consonants. You can refer back to Table 3.2, the Most Common Sounds Pronunciation Key, for assistance with the correct sounds.

Pronounced correctly: The sounds must be pronounced correctly in isolation or blended into words.

Self-corrections: Sounds or words mispronounced initially but corrected within 3 seconds are scored as correct and *sc* is written above the word or if using the computer screen the word is clicked on again to remove the highlighting.

Dialect/articulation: Variations in pronunciation explainable by local language norms or speech sound production.

Repetitions: Repeating the word more than once.

(continued on other side)

Scored as Errors

All errors are marked by drawing a slash through the word or clicking on the word so that it is highlighted with the computer version.

Mispronunciations/substitutions: Letter sounds or words either mispronounced or substituted with other letter sounds.

Omissions: Letter sounds or words that are not produced.

Hesitations without response: Not responding for 3 seconds and being prompted by providing the sound or word.

Hesitations with response: Starting to respond but not finishing by 3 seconds and being prompted by providing the sound or word.

Reversals: Transposing two or more sounds or words.

QUICK ADMINISTRATION GUIDE FOR WORD IDENTIFICATION CBM

1. Place the copy of the student list in front of the student.
2. Place the teacher/examiner copy on the clipboard so the student cannot see it.
3. Say: ***"When I say 'Begin,' I want you to read these words as quickly and correctly as you can. Start here*** (*point to the first word*) ***and go down the page*** (*run your finger down the first column*). ***If you don't know a word, skip it and try the next word. Keep reading until I say 'Stop.' Do you have any questions? Begin."*** (*Trigger stopwatch or timer for 1 minute.*)
4. Follow along on the teacher/examiner copy as the student reads and *put a slash (/) through any incorrect words*.
5. At the end of 1 minute, say: ***"Stop"*** and put a bracket ( ]) after the last word read.

Adapted with permission from Fuchs and Fuchs (2004).

QUICK SCORING GUIDE FOR WORD IDENTIFICATION CBM

Scored as Correct

Word Identification CBM is scored based on the correct pronunciation of the entire word.

Pronounced correctly: The word must be pronounced correctly.

Self-corrections within 3 seconds: Words mispronounced initially but corrected within 3 seconds.

Dialect/articulation: Variations in pronunciation explainable by local language norms or speech sound production.

Repetitions: Repeating the word more than once.

Scored as Errors

All errors are marked with a slash (/) through the word.

Mispronunciations/substitutions: Words either mispronounced or substituted with other words.

Omissions: Words that are not produced.

Hesitations without response: Not responding for 2 seconds and being prompted by pointing to the next word and saying ***"What word?"***

Hesitations with response: Starting to respond but not finishing by 5 seconds and being prompted by pointing to the next word and saying ***"What word?"***

Reversals: Transposes two or more words.

QUICK ADMINISTRATION GUIDE FOR OPR CBM

1. Place the copy of the student passage in front of the student.
2. Place the teacher/examiner copy on the clipboard so the student cannot see it.
3. Say: *"When I say 'Begin,' start reading aloud at the top of the page. Read across the page* (*point to the first line of the passage*). *Try to read each word. If you come to a word you don't know, I'll tell it to you. Be sure to do your best reading. Do you have any questions? Begin."* (*Trigger stopwatch or timer for 1 minute.*)
4. Follow along on the teacher/examiner copy as the student reads and put a slash (/) through any incorrect words.
5. At the end of 1 minute, say *"Thank You"* and mark the last word read with a bracket (]).

_____
Adapted with permission from Shinn (1989)

QUICK SCORING GUIDE FOR OPR CBM

Scored as Correct

OPR CBM is scored based on each word being read accurately within the context of the sentence. Having a black-and-white scoring process increases the reliability of scores between students and assists in ensuring the process remains manageable but still provides good data for each student.

Pronounced correctly: A word must be pronounced correctly, in accordance with the context of the sentence.

Self-corrections within 3 seconds: Words misread initially but corrected within 3 seconds.

Dialect/articulation: Variations in pronunciation explainable by local language norms or speech sound production.

Repetitions: Repeating the same word more than once.

Insertions: Adding extra words to the story.

Scored as Errors

All errors are marked with a slash (/) through the word.

Mispronunciations/word substitutions: When a word is either mispronounced or substituted with another word.

Omissions: Words that are not spoken.

Hesitations without response: Not responding for 3 seconds and being prompted by having the word read.

Hesitations with response: Starting to respond but not finishing by 3 seconds and being prompted by having the word read.

Reversals: Transposing two or more words.

QUICK ADMINISTRATION GUIDE FOR MAZE CBM WITH PRACTICE ITEMS

1. Place a copy of the student passage with the practice items in front of each student (see Figure 4.5 for an example of the practice items).

2. Say: *"Today I want you to read a short story. The story you will read has some places where you will need to choose the correct word. Read the story. When you come to three words in dark print, choose the word that belongs in the sentence.*

   "We will do some examples. Look at the first page. Read the sentence. The sentence says: 'Bill threw the ball to Jane. Jane caught the (dog, bat, ball).' Which one of the three words belongs in the sentence?"

3. After the students respond, say: *"The word 'ball' belongs in the sentence 'Bill threw the ball to Jane. Jane caught the ball.' Circle the word 'ball.'"*

4. *"Now let's try sentence number 2. Read the sentence. The sentence says: 'Tom said, "Now you (jump, throw, talk) the ball to me."' Which of the three words belongs in the sentence?"*

5. After the students respond, say: *"The word 'throw' belongs in the sentence 'Now you throw the ball to me.' Circle the word 'throw.'"*

6. Place a copy of the student passage in front of each student face down.

(continued on other side)

---

7. Say: *"Now you are going to do the same thing by yourself. You will read a story for 1 minute. When I say 'Stop,' stop reading. Do not begin reading until I tell you to start. Whenever you come to three words that are in dark print, circle the word that belongs in the sentence.*

   "Choose a word even if you're not sure of the answer. At the end of 1 minute, I will say 'Stop.' If you finish early, check your answers. Do not go on to the next page. You may turn your paper over and begin when I say 'Start.' Are there any questions?

   "Remember to do the best you can. Pick up your pencils. Ready? Start." (*Trigger stopwatch or timer for 1 minute.*)

8. Walk around the room to monitor students and make sure they are only circling one word per set and not skipping around the page.

9. At the end of 1 minute, say: *"Stop. Put your pencils down."*

10. Separately administer two more passages using the following directions.

11. Say: *"Now you will do the same thing with another story. Remember to choose the word that belongs in the sentence. Choose a word even if you're not sure of the answer. You may begin when I tell you to."* (*Trigger stopwatch or timer for 1 minute.*)

12. At the end of 1 minute, say: *"Stop. Put your pencils down."*

13. Collect all the students' sheets.

Adapted with permission from Edcheckup (2005).

QUICK ADMINISTRATION GUIDE FOR MAZE CBM
WITHOUT PRACTICE ITEMS

1. Place a copy of the student passage in front of each student face down. (It is helpful to have the student's name already on the sheet before starting.)

2. Say: ***"When I say 'Begin,' turn to the first story and start reading silently. When you come to a group of three words, circle the one word that makes the most sense. Work as quickly as you can without making mistakes. If you finish the page, turn the page and keep working until I say 'Stop' or you are all done. Do you have any questions? Begin."*** (*Trigger stopwatch or timer for 3 minutes.*)

3. Walk around the room to monitor students and make sure they are only circling one word per set and not skipping around the page.

4. At the end of 3 minutes, say: ***"Stop. Put your pencil down and turn your sheet over."***

5. Collect all the students' sheets.

Adapted with permission from aimsweb (Shinn & Shinn, 2002b).

QUICK SCORING GUIDE FOR MAZE CBM

Scored as Correct

Maze CBM is scored based on the student picking the correct word to restore the meaning to the sentence. The student must circle or underline his choice.

Answered correctly: The correct word is circled or underlined.

Scored as Errors

All errors are marked by putting a slash (/) through the correct choice if the incorrect word is circled, underlined, or left blank.

QUICK ADMINISTRATION GUIDE FOR SPELLING CBM

1. Select an appropriate grade-level spelling list.
2. Have students number their papers from 1 to 12 for first and second graders or 1 to 17 for third grade and up.
3. Say: *"I am going to read some words to you. I want you to write the words on the sheet in front of you. Write the first word on the first line, the second word on the second line, and so on. I'll give you 10 seconds [7 seconds for grade 3 and up] to spell each word. When I say the next word, try to write it, even if you haven't finished the last one. Are there any questions?"*
4. Say the first word and trigger stopwatch or timer for 2 minutes.
5. Say each word twice. Use homonyms in a sentence.
6. Say a new word every 10 seconds (grades 1 and 2) or 7 seconds (grade 3 and up).
7. At the end of 2 minutes, say: *"Thank you. Put your pencils down."*

_____

Adapted with permission from Shinn (1989).

QUICK SCORING GUIDE FOR SPELLING CBM

Scoring Correct Letter Sequences (CLS)

CLS is the number of correct sequences related to spelling, the space before and after the word, and the letter to punctuation (before and after). When scoring CLS, the scorer places a caret (^) to indicate each correct sequence.

Compound words: Words need to stay together without a space.

Apostrophe: The spaces before and after an apostrophe are counted.

Hyphens: The spaces before and after a hyphen are counted.

Capitalization: A word that should be capitalized must begin with a capital letter.

Repeated letters in sequence: Words with letters that are repeated in sequence are scored the same as if each letter were different.

Additional letters: Additional letters are not counted twice.

Insertions: Extra letters at the beginning and end are not counted.

QUICK ADMINISTRATION GUIDE FOR WRITING CBM

1. Provide students with a pencil and piece of lined paper or writing notebook.
2. Select an appropriate story starter.
3. Say: *"Today I want you to write a story. I am going to read a sentence to you first and then I want you to compose a short story about what happens. You will have 1 minute to think about what you will write and 3 minutes to write your story. Remember to do your best work. If you do not know how to spell a word, you should guess. Are there any questions?"* (*Pause*) **Put your pencils down and listen. For the next minute, think about** . . . (*insert story starter*)."
4. After reading the story starter, begin your stopwatch and allow 1 minute for the student(s) to think. (*Monitor students so that they do not begin writing.*) After 30 seconds say: *"You should be thinking about . . .* (*insert story starter*)." At the end of 1 minute, restart your stopwatch for 3 minutes and say: *"Now begin writing."*
5. Monitor students' attention to the task. Encourage the students to work if they are not writing.
6. After 90 seconds say: *"You should be writing about . . .* (*insert story starter*)."
7. At the end of 3 minutes say: *"Thank you. Put your pencils down."*

_____

Adapted with permission from aimsweb (Powell-Smith & Shinn, 2004).

QUICK SCORING GUIDE FOR WRITING CBM:
TOTAL WORDS WRITTEN (TWW)

TWW is the number of words written regardless of spelling or context. When scoring TWW, the scorer underlines each word written and records the total number of words written (see Figure 6.3). Words are defined as any letter or group of letters, including misspelled or nonsense words, that have a space before and after them.

Abbreviations: Common abbreviations are counted as words (e.g., Dr., Mrs., TV).

Hyphenated words: Each morpheme in a hyphenated word separated by a hyphen is counted as an individual word if it can stand alone. Prefixes separated by a hyphen are not counted as words, although the root word is counted.

Titles and endings: Story titles and endings are counted as words written.

Numerals: Numerals, with the exception of dates and currency, are not counted as words unless they are written out (i.e., as words).

Unusual characters: Unusual characters are not counted as words even if they are meant to take the place of a word.

QUICK SCORING GUIDE FOR WRITING CBM: WORDS SPELLED CORRECTLY (WSC)

WSC is the number of correctly spelled words, regardless of context. Words are counted in WSC if they can be found in the English language. Incorrectly spelled words should be circled (see Figure 6.3). WSC is calculated by subtracting the total number of circled words from the TWW. As with TWW, additional scoring rules apply to WSC.

Abbreviations: Abbreviations must be spelled correctly.

Hyphenated words: Each morpheme counted as an individual word must be spelled correctly. If the morpheme cannot stand alone (e.g., prefix) and part of the word is incorrect, the entire word is counted as an incorrect spelling.

Titles and endings: Words in the title or ending are counted in the words spelled correctly.

Capitalization: Proper nouns must be capitalized unless the name is also a common noun. Capitalization of the first word in the sentence is not a requirement for the word to be spelled correctly. Words are counted as spelled correctly even if they are capitalized incorrectly within the sentence.

Reversed letters: Words containing letter reversals are not counted as errors unless the reversal causes the word to be spelled incorrectly. This typically applies with reversals of the following letters: *p, q, g, d, b, n, u.*

Contractions: In order for a contraction to be counted as correct, it must have the apostrophe in the correct place unless the word can stand alone.

QUICK SCORING GUIDE FOR WRITING CBM: CORRECT WRITING SEQUENCES (CWS)

A CWS is "two adjacent, correctly spelled words that are acceptable within the context of the [written] phrase to a native speaker of the English language" (Videen et al., 1982, p. 7). It takes into account punctuation, syntax, semantics, spelling, and capitalization. When scoring CWS, a caret (^) is used to mark each correct word sequence. A space is implied at the beginning of a sentence. The following should be taken into consideration when scoring CWS.

Spelling: Words must be spelled correctly to be counted in CWS. Words that are not counted in WSC or are circled words are *not* counted as correct writing sequences.

Capitalization: Capitalization at the beginning of the sentence is necessary. Proper nouns must be capitalized unless they can serve as common nouns in the given context. Incorrectly capitalized words are marked as incorrect CWS.

Punctuation: Punctuation at the end of the sentence must be correct. Commas are not typically counted unless they are used in a series. In a series, they must be used correctly to be scored. Other punctuation marks are typically not counted as CWS.

Syntax: Words must be syntactically correct to be counted as CWS. Sentences that begin with a conjunction are considered to be syntactically correct.

Semantics: Words must be semantically correct to be counted in CWS.

Story titles and endings: Story titles and endings are included in the scoring of CWS and must meet scoring criteria for spelling, punctuation, capitalization, syntax, and semantics to be counted in CWS.

QUICK ADMINISTRATION GUIDE FOR ORAL COUNTING CBM

1. Place the teacher/examiner copy on the clipboard so the student cannot see it.
2. Say: *"When I say 'Start' I want you to start counting aloud from 1, like this: 1, 2, 3, until I tell you to stop. If you come to a number you don't know, I'll tell it to you. Be sure to do your best counting. Ready? Start."* (*Trigger timer for 1 minute.*)
3. Follow along on the teacher/examiner copy as the student counts and put a slash (/) through any incorrect or skipped numbers.
4. At the end of 1 minute say *"Stop"* and put a bracket (]) after the last number counted.

_____

Adapted with permission from aimsweb (Shinn & Shinn, 2002a).

QUICK ADMINISTRATION GUIDE FOR TOUCH COUNTING CBM

1. Place a copy of the student sheet in front of the student.
2. Place the teacher/examiner copy on the clipboard so the student cannot see it.
3. Say: *"When I say 'Begin' I want you to start counting from the top of the page* (*point to the first dot*) *until I tell you to stop. Count across the page. When you come to the end of a row, go to the next row. If you come to a number you don't know, I'll tell it to you. Be sure to do your best counting. Ready? Begin."* (*Trigger timer for 1 minute.*)
4. Follow along on the teacher/examiner copy as the student counts and put a slash (/) through any incorrect or skipped numbers.
5. At the end of 1 minute say: *"Please stop"* and put a bracket (]) after the last number counted.

_____

QUICK SCORING GUIDE FOR ORAL AND TOUCH COUNTING CBM

Scored as Correct

Oral Counting CBM and Touch Counting CBM are scored based on each number that is stated correctly or touched correctly as it is associated with a correct number amount. Each correct response counts toward the total score defined as the total number correct (NC).

Pronounced/answered correctly: A number must be correctly pronounced in the correct order. For Touch Counting CBM, it also must be associated with the pointing to or touching of one circle.

Self-corrections within 3 seconds: Numbers miscounted initially but corrected within 3 seconds are scored as correct. If already slashed as an error, the number is circled.

Dialect/articulation: Variations in pronunciation explainable by local language norms or speech sound production.

Repetitions: Repeating the same number(s) more than once before moving on.

Insertions: Adding a number that does not belong in the sequence.

(continued)

Scored as Errors

All errors are marked with a slash (/) through the number.

Mispronunciations/substitutions: When a nonnumber name or name of wrong number is given.

Omissions: Numbers that are not produced.

Hesitations without response: Not responding for 3 seconds and being prompted by providing the number.

Hesitations with response: Starting to respond but not finishing within 3 seconds and being prompted by providing the number.

Reversals: Transposing two or more numbers.

Skipped items: A number is skipped in a sequence and not stated.

QUICK ADMINISTRATION GUIDE FOR NUMBER IDENTIFICATION CBM

1. Place the student copy in front of the student.
2. Place the teacher/examiner copy on the clipboard so the student cannot see it.
3. Say: **"Look at the paper in front of you. There are numbers in boxes** (point to the first box). **What number is this?"**
   a. If student gives the correct response, say: **"Good. The number is 6."** (Point to the second box.)
   b. If the student gives an incorrect response, say: **"This number is 6. What number?"** (Point to the second box.)
4. Continue with the other example(s). After the examples, turn to the first page of the student copy of the sheets.
5. Say: **"When I say begin, I want you to tell me what number is in each box. Start here and go across the page** (demonstrate by pointing). **Try each one. If you come to one that you don't know, I'll tell you what to do. Are there any questions? Put your finger on the first one. Ready? Begin."** (Trigger timer for 1 minute.)
6. On the administrator copy, write the number that the student says in the blank next to each problem number.
7. If the student comes to the end of the page, turn the page to the next page of numbers.
8. At the end of 1 minute, draw a bracket ( ]) after the last item completed and say **"Stop."**

_____

Adapted with permission from Research Institute on Progress Monitoring.

QUICK SCORING GUIDE FOR NUMBER IDENTIFICATION CBM

Scored as Correct

Number Identification CBM is scored based on each number that is stated correctly as it is associated with a correct number amount. Each correct response counts toward the total score defined as the total number correct (NC).

Pronounced/answered correctly: The name of each number must be correctly pronounced in the correct order.

Self-corrections within 3 seconds: Numbers misidentified initially but corrected within 3 seconds.

Dialect/articulation: Variations in pronunciation explainable by local language norms or speech sound production.

Repetitions: Repeating the same number(s) more than once before moving on.

Insertions: Adding numbers that are not on the stimulus sheet.

Scored as Errors

All errors are marked with a slash (/).

Mispronunciations/substitutions: When a nonnumber name or name of wrong number is given.

Omissions: Numbers that are not produced.

Hesitations without response: Not responding for 3 seconds and being prompted by providing the number.

Hesitations with response: Starting to respond but not finishing by 3 seconds and being prompted by providing the number.

Skipped items: A number is skipped in a sequence and not stated.

QUICK ADMINISTRATION GUIDE FOR MISSING NUMBER CBM

1. Place the student copy in front of the student.
2. Place the teacher/examiner copy on the clipboard so the student cannot see it.
3. Say: *"Look at the paper in front of you. Each box has three numbers and a blank* (point to the first box). *What number goes in the blank?"*
   a. If student gives a correct response, say: *"Good. The number is 3."* (Point to the second box.)
   b. If the student gives an incorrect response, *"The number that goes in the blank is 3. You should have said 3 because 3 comes after 2 (0, 1, 2, 3)."* (Point to the second box.)
4. Continue with the other example(s). After the examples, turn to the first page of the student copy of the sheets.
5. Say: *"When I say begin, I want you to tell me what number goes in the blank in each box. Start here and go across the page* (demonstrate by pointing). *Try each one. If you come to one that you don't know, I'll tell you what to do. Are there any questions? Put your finger on the first one. Ready? Begin."* (Trigger timer for 1 minute.)
6. On the administrator copy, write the number that the student says in the blank next to each problem number.
7. If the student comes to the end of the page, turn the page to the next page of problems.
8. At the end of 1 minute, draw a bracket ( ]) after the last item completed and say *"Stop."*

———

Adapted with permission from Research Institute on Progress Monitoring.

QUICK SCORING GUIDE FOR MISSING NUMBER CBM

Scored as Correct

Missing Number CBM is scored based on each correct number identified that completes the number pattern. Each correct response counts toward the total score defined as the total number correct (NC).

Pronounced/answered correctly: The name of the appropriate number to complete the pattern must be correctly pronounced.

Self-corrections within 3 seconds: Numbers misidentified initially but corrected within 3 seconds are scored as correct.

Dialect/articulation: Variations in pronunciation explainable by local language norms or speech sound production are correct.

Scored as Errors

All errors are marked with a slash (/).

Mispronunciations/substitutions: When a nonnumber name or name of wrong number is used.

Hesitations without response: Not responding for 3 seconds and being prompted by moving on to the next item.

Hesitations with response: Starting to respond but not finishing by 3 seconds and being prompted by moving on to the next item.

QUICK ADMINISTRATION GUIDE FOR QUANTITY DISCRIMINATION CBM

1. Place the student copy in front of the student.

2. Place the teacher/examiner copy on the clipboard so the student cannot see it.

3. Say: ***"Look at the paper in front of you. In each row there are some boxes with numbers in them"*** (point to the first box). ***"I want you to tell me the number that is bigger."***

   a. If the student gives the correct response, say: ***"Good. 7 is bigger than 1."*** (Point to the second box.)

   b. If the student gives an incorrect response, say: ***"The number that is bigger is 7. You should have said 7 because 7 is bigger than 1."*** (Point to the second box.)

4. Continue with the other example(s). After the examples, turn to the first page of the student copy of the sheets.

5. Say: ***"When I say begin, I want you to tell me which number is bigger. Start here and go across the page*** (demonstrate by pointing). ***Try each one. If you come to one that you don't know, I'll tell you what to do. Are there any questions? Put your finger on the first one. Ready? Begin."*** (Trigger timer for 1 minute.)

6. On the administrator copy, write the number that the student says in the blank next to each problem number.

7. If the student comes to the end of the page, turn the page to the next page of problems.

8. At the end of 1 minute, draw a bracket ( ]) after the last item completed and say ***"Stop."***

_____

Adapted with permission from Research Institute on Progress Monitoring.

QUICK SCORING GUIDE FOR QUANTITY DISCRIMINATION CBM

Scored as Correct

Quantity Discrimination CBM is scored based on each correct response the student gives that indicates the bigger number. Each correct response counts toward the total score defined as the total number correct (NC).

Pronounced/answered correctly: The name of the appropriate larger number must be correctly pronounced.

Self-corrections within 3 seconds: Numbers misidentified initially but corrected within 3 seconds.

Dialect/articulation: Variations in pronunciation explainable by local language norms or speech sound production.

Scored as Errors

All errors are marked with a slash (/).

Mispronunciations/substitutions: When a nonnumber name or name of a wrong number is used.

Hesitations without response: Not responding for 3 seconds and being prompted to move to the next item.

Hesitations with response: Starting to respond but not finishing by 3 seconds and being prompted to move to the next item.

Skipped items: A number that is skipped in a sequence.

QUICK ADMINISTRATION GUIDE FOR M-COMP CBM (SINGLE OPERATION)

1. Place a copy of the student sheet in front of the students.
2. For single-operation sheets, say: ***"The sheets on your desk have*** (*addition, subtraction, multiplication, division, fractions, ratios, decimals, etc.*) ***problems on them. Look at each problem carefully before you answer it. When I say, 'Please begin,' start answering the problems. Begin with the first problem and work across the page*** (*point*). ***Then go to the next row. If you cannot answer the problem, mark an 'X' through it and go to the next one. If you finish a page, turn the page and continue working until I say 'Thank you.' Are there any questions? Please begin."***
3. Once you say ***"Please begin,"*** start the countdown timer (*set for 2 minutes or the appropriate time limit*). At the end of the time limit, say ***"Thank you"*** and have the students put their pencils down and stop working.

Adapted with permission from Shinn (1989).

QUICK ADMINISTRATION GUIDE FOR M-COMP CBM (MIXED OPERATION)

1. Place a copy of the student sheet in front of the students.
2. For mixed-operation sheets, say: ***"The sheets on your desk have math problems on them. There are several types of problems on the sheet. Some are*** (*insert types of problems on sheet*). ***Look at each problem carefully before you answer it. When I say 'Please begin,' start answering the problems. Begin with the first problem and work across the page*** (*point*). ***Then go to the next row. If you cannot answer the problem, mark an 'X' through it and go to the next one. If you finish a page, turn the page and continue working until I say 'Thank you.' Are there any questions? Please begin."***
3. Once you say ***"Please begin,"*** start the countdown timer (*set for 2 minutes or the appropriate time limit*). At the end of the time limit, say ***"Thank you"*** and have the students put their pencils down and stop working.

Adapted with permission from Shinn (1989).

QUICK SCORING GUIDE FOR M-COMP CBM

Scored as Correct

Answered correctly: If the student has the correct answer, she is given credit for 1 CP, the number of CD in the answer (CD-A), or the longest method used to solve the problem *even if all the work is not shown* (for CD-S). If the student gets the correct answer, she has demonstrated that she knows how to solve the problem and, therefore, gets full credit in whichever metric is used.

Incomplete/crossed out: If a problem has been crossed out or started, but not completed, the student still receives appropriate credit. Correct work is correct work, even if the student did not finish the problem.

Reversed/rotated: Reversed or rotated digits are scored as correct with the exception of 6's and 9's. With 6's and 9's, it is not possible to tell which one the student meant to write. No other digits can become others through rotation or reversal.

Placeholder: In multiplication problems, any symbol used as a placeholder is counted as a correct digit as long as it is holding a place that needs to be held. The student can use a 0, X, ☺, a blank space, or whatever else as long as it is used to hold that place.

(continued)

Scored as Errors

All errors are marked with a slash (/). See Figure 8.4 (panels D, E, and F) for three examples.

Substitutions: When the student writes the wrong number.
Omissions: Each number omitted is an error.

QUICK ADMINISTRATION GUIDE FOR M-CAP CBM

1. Place a copy of the student sheet in front of the students.

2. Say: *"The sheets on your desk have math problems on them. There are several types of math problems on the sheet. Look at each problem carefully before you answer it. When I say 'Please begin,' start answering the problems. Begin with the first problem and work in the order presented* (point). *If you cannot answer the problem, mark an 'X' through it and go to the next one. If you finish a page, turn the page and continue working until I say 'Thank you.' Are there any questions? Please begin."*

3. Once you say **"Please begin,"** start the countdown timer (*set for 6 minutes or the appropriate time limit*). At the end of the time limit, say: **"Thank you"** and have the students put their pencils down and stop working.

Adapted with permission from Shinn (1989).

QUICK SCORING GUIDE FOR M-CAP CBM

Scored as Correct

Answered correctly: Some publishers still use a production response (adhering to original CBM principles) such that the student needs to produce the response she thinks is correct by writing it in a blank. If this is the case, the student's response must be compared to that in the answer key. For the sake of simplicity and greater automation, some publishers are using a selected response format (i.e., multiple choice with three potential responses). This is a simplified format for computerized administration advances. Although within a framework of instructional hierarchy or Bloom's taxonomy this represents a different level of mastery of the task, preliminary research suggests similar technical adequacy. Given the savings in time for administration and scoring, this could increase utility of the measures. If the student has the correct answer, she is given credit for 1 CP, which will be converted to a predetermined number of points (generally 1–3) using a table in the scoring manual.

Incomplete/crossed out: If a problem has been crossed out or started, but not completed, the student still receives appropriate credit. Correct work is correct work, even if the student did not finish the problem.

Reversed/rotated: Reversed or rotated digits are scored as correct with the exception of 6's and 9's. With 6's and 9's, it is not possible to tell which one the student meant to write. No other digits can become others through rotation or reversal.

Scored as Errors

All errors are marked with a slash (/). See Figure 8.4 (panels D, E, and F) for three examples.

Substitutions: When a student writes the wrong number.

Omissions: Each number that is not recorded.

QUICK ADMINISTRATION GUIDE FOR VOCABULARY MATCHING CBM

1. Place the student copy in front of the student(s).
2. Say: *"Look at the paper in front of you. There are vocabulary words on the left* (point to the column of vocabulary words) *and definitions for those words are on the right* (point to the column of definitions). *The definitions are in a mixed-up order, but every vocabulary word has its appropriate definition in the right column."*
3. Say: *"When I say begin, I want you to write the letter of the definition in the blank in front of the appropriate vocabulary word* (demonstrate by pointing). *Try each one. If you come to one that you don't know, you can come back to it. Are there any questions? Begin."* (Trigger timer for 5 minutes.)
4. If the student comes to the end of the page, make sure he continues working until the time is up.
5. At the end of 5 minutes, say *"Stop."*

QUICK SCORING GUIDE FOR VOCABULARY MATCHING CBM

Scored as Correct

Letter representing the correct definition for the vocabulary term.

Scored as Errors

Letter representing an incorrect definition for the vocabulary term.
Letter representing a distractor definition.

GRAPH FOR PROGRESS MONITORING DATA

Student: _____   Teacher: _____   Grade: _____   Level: _____

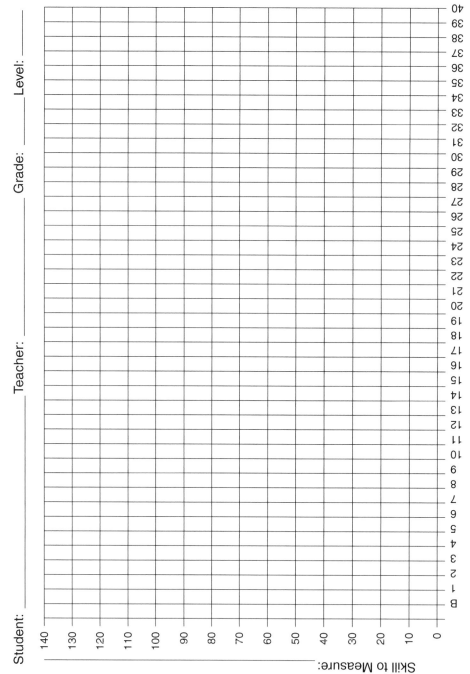

Skill to Measure:

Weeks

CHECKLIST FOR USING CBM BEFORE, DURING, AND AFTER INITIAL IMPLEMENTATION

BEFORE

Step 1: Who will be using CBM? (Check all that apply.)

____ Classroom(s)   ____ Grade(s)   ____ School(s)   ____ District

Step 2: Which CBM skills will be measured? (Check all that apply.)

Early Reading	____	Onset Sounds
	____	Phoneme Segmenting
	____	Letter Naming
	____	Letter Sounds
	____	Nonsense Words
	____	Word Identification
Reading	____	Oral Passage Reading
	____	Maze
Spelling	____	CLS (correct letter sequences)
	____	WSC (words spelled correctly)
Writing	____	TWW (total words written)
	____	WSC (words spelled correctly)
	____	CWS (correct writing sequences)
Early Numeracy	____	Oral Counting
	____	Touch Counting
	____	Number Identification
	____	Missing Number
	____	Quantity Discrimination
Math	____	Computation (mixed operation)
	____	Computation (single operation)
	____	Concepts and Applications
Vocabulary	____	Matching

Step 3: What materials will we use?

____ Use a commercial product with administration, scoring, and graphing program

____ Purchase premade material (i.e., pastsages, lists, sheets, story starters) and make your own graphing program

____ Purchase premade materials (i.e., passages, lists, sheets, story starters) and graph on paper

Step 4: When will implementation start?

____ Fall   ____ Winter   ____ Spring

(continued)

Step 5: Who will train the staff?

_____ Hire a professional trainer to train the staff

_____ Have a couple of staff members receive professional training and then train the rest of the staff

_____ Train yourselves by using published materials and practicing together as a group

DURING

Step 6: Who will manage the materials?

_____ Teacher (general education, Title I, ESL, special education)

_____ Administrator (principal, vice principal)

_____ Support staff (speech therapist, reading specialist, school psychologist)

_____ Assistants (administrative assistants, parent volunteers)

Step 7: Who will collect the data?

_____ Individual teachers

_____ Teams (e.g., general and special education teachers, educational assistants, principals, school psychologists, reading specialists, speech therapists)

Step 8: Where will the data be collected?

_____ In the classroom

_____ Central location (library, cafeteria, multipurpose room)

AFTER

Step 9: Who will manage the data once they are collected?

_____ Each teacher is responsible for entering and graphing students' data

_____ One person for each grade or school is responsible for entering and graphing the data

_____ A team of people at the district level is responsible for entering and graphing the data

Step 10: How will the data be shared? (check all that apply)

_____ Each teacher is responsible for looking at his or her own data

_____ At the grade level, all of the teachers look at all of the students together

_____ At the school level, a team is responsible for looking at all of the students

GENERAL FIDELITY CHECKLIST FOR CONDUCTING CBM

BEFORE

Yes   No

☐   ☐   1. Has the correct student material and teacher/examiner material.

☐   ☐   2. Has the appropriate device to mark students' responses (computer or pen/pencil).

☐   ☐   3. Has the appropriate timing device (computer or countdown timer).

☐   ☐   4. Positions the computer screen or clipboard so student cannot see scoring.

DURING

Yes   No

☐   ☐   5. Reads the standardized directions verbatim.

☐   ☐   6. Starts the timer according to the directions.

☐   ☐   7. Follows the procedure for time allowed on each item.

☐   ☐   8. Marks the student's errors on an appropriate device (computer or teacher/examiner sheet).

☐   ☐   9. Does not correct the student when he or she makes an error (except when allowed in the example material and only then).

☐   ☐   10. Follows the discontinuation rule.

☐   ☐   11. Administers the task for the correct amount of time.

☐   ☐   12. Stops the student at the end of the time and marks where the student stops.

AFTER

Yes   No

☐   ☐   13. Submits the completed assessment via computer

or

☐   ☐   14. Adds up the total number of items attempted correctly.

☐   ☐   15. Adds up the total number of errors correctly.

☐   ☐   16. Calculates the rate score correctly.

☐   ☐   17. Calculates the accuracy score correctly.

☐   ☐   18. Prorates the score if the student finishes the task before the time is up.

☐   ☐   19. Graphs the score correctly.

References

Coker, D. L., & Ritchey, K. D. (2010). Curriculum-based measurement of writing in kindergarten and first grade: An investigation of production and qualitative scores. *Exceptional Children, 76,* 175–193.

Deno, S. L. (2003). Developments in curriculum-based measurement. *Journal of Special Education, 37,* 184–192.

Deno, S. L., Marston, D., & Mirkin, P. K. (1982). Valid measurement procedures for continuous evaluation of written expression. *Exceptional Children, 48,* 368–371.

Deno, S. L., & Mirkin, P. K. (1977). *Data-based program modification: A manual.* Reston, VA: Council for Exceptional Children.

Deno, S. L., Mirkin, P. K., Lowry, L., & Kuehnle, K. (1980). *Relationships among simple measures of spelling and performance on standardized tests* (Research Report No. 21). Minneapolis: University of Minnesota, Institute for Research on Learning Disabilities.

Edcheckup. (2005). *Administering the oral reading CBM assessment* [section 2]. Minneapolis, MN: Author.

Espin, C. A., Scierka, B. J., Skare, S., & Halverson, N. (1999). Criterion-related validity of curriculum-based measures in writing for secondary school students. *Reading and Writing Quarterly: Overcoming Learning Difficulties, 15*(1), 5–27.

Espin, C. A., Shin, J., Deno, S. L., Skare, S., Robinson, S., & Benner, B. (2000). Identifying indicators of written expression proficiency for middle school students. *Journal of Special Education, 34,* 140–153.

Fuchs, L. S., & Fuchs, D. (1991). Curriculum-based measurements: Current applications and future directions. *Preventing School Failure, 35*(3), 6–11.

Fuchs, L. S., & Fuchs, D. (2004). Using CBM for progress monitoring. Retrieved from *www.studentprogress.org.*

Fuchs, L. S., Fuchs, D., & Hamlett, C. L. (1989). Computers and curriculum-based measurement: Effect of teacher feedback systems. *School Psychology Review, 18,* 112–125.

Fuchs, L. S., Fuchs, D., Hamlett, C. L., Walz, L., & Germann, G. (1993). Formative evaluation of academic progress: How much growth can we expect? *School Psychology Review, 22,* 27–49.

Fuchs, L. S., Fuchs, D., Hosp, M. K., & Jenkins, J. (2001). Oral reading fluency as an indicator of reading competence: A theoretical, empirical, and historical analysis. *Journal for the Society of the Scientific Study of Reading, 5,* 239–256.

Gansle, K. A., Noell, G. H., VanDerHeyden, A. M., Naquin, G. M., & Slider, N. J. (2002). Moving beyond total words written: The reliability, criterion validity, and time cost of alternate measures for curriculum-based measurement in writing. *School Psychology Review, 31,* 477–497.

Hosp, J. L., Hosp, M. K., Howell, K. W., & Allison, R. (2014). *The ABCs of curriculum-based evaluation: A practical guide to effective decision making.* New York: Guilford Press.

Jimerson, S., Burns, M., & VanDerHeyden, A. (Eds.). (2016). *Handbook of response to intervention: The science and practice of assessment and intervention* (2nd ed.). New York: Springer.

Lembke, E., Deno, S. L., & Hall, K. (2003). Identifying an indicator of growth in early writing proficiency for elementary school students. *Assessment for Effective Intervention, 28,* 23–35.

Loeffler, K. A. (2005). No more Friday spelling test? *Teaching Exceptional Children, 37*(4), 24–27.

Malecki, C. K., & Jewell, J. (2003). Developmental, gender, and practical considerations in scoring curriculum-based writing probes. *Psychology in the Schools, 40,* 379–390.

McMaster, K. L., Du, X., & Petursdottir, A. (2009). Technical features of curriculum-based measures for beginning writers. *Journal of Learning Disabilities, 42,* 41–60.

Methe, S., Begeny, J., & Leary, L. (2011). Development of conceptually focused early numeracy skill indicators. *Assessment for Effective Intervention, 36,* 230–242.

National Council for Teachers of Mathematics. (2000). *Principles and standards for school mathematics.* Reston, VA: Author.

National Governors Association Center for Best Practices & Council of Chief State School Officers. (2010). *Common Core State Standards.* Washington, DC: Authors.

National Institute of Child Health and Human Development. (2000, April). *Report of the National Reading Panel: Teaching children to read.* Washington, DC: Author.

National Mathematics Advisory Panel. (2008). *Foundations for success: The final report of the National Mathematics Advisory Panel.* Washington, DC: U.S. Department of Education.

National Research Council. (1998). *Preventing reading difficulties in young children.* Washington, DC: National Academy Press.

Powell-Smith, K. A., & Shinn, M. R. (2004). *Administration and scoring of written expression curriculum-based measurement for use in general outcome measurement.* Eden Prairie, MN: Edformation.

Riley-Tillman, T., & Burns, M. (2009). *Evaluating educational interventions: Single-case design for measuring response to intervention.* New York: Guilford Press.

Ritchey, K. D. (2006). Learning to write: Progress-monitoring tools for beginning and at-risk writers. *Teaching Exceptional Children, 39,* 22–26.

Robbins, K., Hosp, J., Hosp, M., & Flynn, L. (2010). Assessing specific grapho-phonemic skills in elementary students. *Assessment for Effective Intervention, 36,* 21–34.

Shinn, M. R. (1989). *Curriculum-based measurement: Assessing special children.* New York: Guilford Press.

Shinn, M. R., & Shinn, M. M. (2002a). *AIMSweb training workbook: Administration and scoring of early literacy measures for use with AIMSweb.* Eden Prairie, MN: Edformation.

Shinn, M. R., & Shinn, M. M. (2002b). *AIMSweb training workbook: Administration and scoring of reading maze for use in general outcome measurement.* Eden Prairie, MN: Edformation.

Snow, C. E., Burns, M. S., & Griffin, P. (Eds.). (1998). *Preventing reading difficulties in young children.* Washington, DC: National Academy Press.

Vellutino, F. R., Scanlon, D. M., Small, S., & Fanuele, D. P. (2006). Response to intervention as a vehicle for distinguishing between children with and without reading disabilities. *Journal of Learning Disabilities, 39,* 157–169.

Videen, J., Deno, S., & Marston, D. B. (1982). *Correct word sequences: A valid indicator of written expression* (Research Report No. 84). Minneapolis: University of Minnesota Institute for Research on Learning Disabilities.

Watkinson, J. T., & Lee, S. W. (1992). Curriculum-based measures of written expression for learning-disabled and non-disabled students. *Psychology in the Schools, 29,* 184–191.

Index

Note. f or *t* following a page number indicates a figure or a table.